PRAISE FOR *HIGH MAGICK*

"I passed the first seventeen years of my life without so much as a moment of serious self-reflection. A few pleasant puffs from a clumsily rolled joint shared with my dear older brother changed that…changed everything. Cannabis became for me a sacrament, and, quite literally, the gateway to magick. Farber's *High Magick* is a most timely and comprehensive look at the evolutionary and magical potentials of this sacred magical entity."

—Lon Milo DuQuette, author of *Low Magick*

"What an amazing book! A concise yet thorough, well-researched treatise weaving philosophical musings with useful exercises to enhance your enjoyment and utilization of all things cannabis. From dreadlocks to dishabituation, hypnosis to contact highs, I loved how this book kept coming back to the importance of ritual and the art of always being open to possibility. *High Magick* is an important signpost on the road to the entheogenic revolution. Bravo, Phil Farber!"

—Julie Holland, MD, editor of
The Pot Book: A Complete Guide to Cannabis

"Farber has provided us with a well-researched, intelligent, and playful grimoire for initiates of the Herb Dangerous, aka cannabis. From NLP-savvy mind hacks to group ceremonial practice, *High Magick* details the history, pharmacology, and mythology of cannabis and brings it all to life with practical esoteric techniques. Highly recommended indeed!"

—Julian Vayne, author of
Getting Higher: The Manual of Psychedelic Ceremony

"Phil Farber's *High Magick* is an excellent and accessible introduction to the historical role of cannabis in the magical tradition and its practical application by today's modern magicians. Highly recommended."

—Chris Bennett, author of
Liber 420: Cannabis, Magickal Herbs, and the Occult

T0346736

"In the mind-expanding, interdisciplinary tradition of Aleister Crowley and Robert Anton Wilson, Farber explores the powerful interface between magick and the disciplined use of the cannabis plant ... Overflowing with ancient lore, current science, effective exercises, and personal experiences that are at once practical and inspirational. Highly recommended!"

—David Jay Brown, author *Dreaming Wide Awake*
and *The New Science of Psychedelics*

"The magical use of cannabis is known among the Daoists and ancient Scythians. It is also a thread that connects the work of Francois Rabelais, John Dee and Edward Kelley, Paschal Beverly Randolph, Aleister Crowley, and Timothy Leary. Phil Farber's *High Magick* represents a culmination of this lineage in the sense that the powerful and direct 'meta-magick' practices that Farber teaches will help you to further blow those older practices wide open or to entirely create your own—or both!"

—Edward Pandemonium, author of *Twilight Language*
and *The Gospel of Pandemonium*

HIGH MAGICK

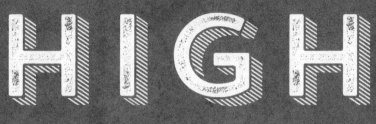

HIGH MAGICK

A GUIDE TO CANNABIS IN RITUAL & MYSTICISM

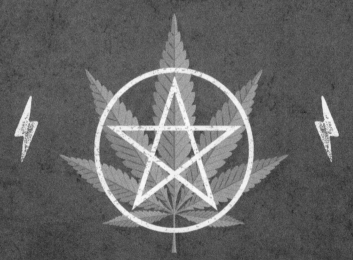

PHILIP H. FARBER

LLEWELLYN PUBLICATIONS
WOODBURY, MINNESOTA

FIRST EDITION
Fifth Printing, 2024

Cover design by Kevin R. Brown
Interior art by the Llewellyn Art Department

Llewellyn Publications is a registered trademark of Llewellyn Worldwide Ltd.

Library of Congress Cataloging-in-Publication Data
Names: Farber, Philip H., author.
Title: High magick : a guide to cannabis in ritual & mysticism / Philip H. Farber.
Description: Woodbury, Minnesota : Llewellyn Publications, 2020. | Includes index.
Identifiers: LCCN 2019055229 (print) | LCCN 2019055230 (ebook) | ISBN 9780738762661 (paperback) | ISBN 9780738763026 (ebook)
Subjects: LCSH: Magic. | Cannabis—Miscellanea. | Occultism. | Hallucinogenic drugs and religious experience.
Classification: LCC BF1623.D74 F37 2020 (print) | LCC BF1623.D74 (ebook) | DDC 133.4/3—dc23
LC record available at https://lccn.loc.gov/2019055229
LC ebook record available at https://lccn.loc.gov/2019055230

Llewellyn Worldwide Ltd. does not participate in, endorse, or have any authority or responsibility concerning private business transactions between our authors and the public.

All mail addressed to the author is forwarded but the publisher cannot, unless specifically instructed by the author, give out an address or phone number.

Any internet references contained in this work are current at publication time, but the publisher cannot guarantee that a specific location will continue to be maintained. Please refer to the publisher's website for links to authors' websites and other sources.

Llewellyn Publications
A Division of Llewellyn Worldwide Ltd.
2143 Wooddale Drive
Woodbury, MN 55125-2989
www.llewellyn.com

Printed in the United States of America

OTHER BOOKS BY PHILIP H. FARBER

Nonfiction

FutureRitual: Magick for the 21st Century
Meta-Magick: The Book of Atem
Brain Magick: Exercises in Meta-Magick and Invocation

Fiction

The Great Purple Hoo-Ha
Legendary Blue Smoke

CONTENTS

INTRODUCTION

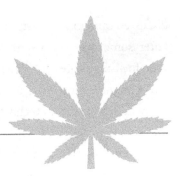

Here in the United States of America, in the early years of the twenty-first century, attitudes and laws about cannabis are changing rapidly. As of this writing, a handful of states have legalized the use of cannabis across the board and dozens more have legalized some form of medical marijuana. Our nation and the world are cautiously lifting the blinders of prohibition and rediscovering the history and uses of this remarkable plant.

Some of us are starting to speak out about the various ways that cannabis has helped and influenced us over the years. We are starting to hear stories of medical patients who find that cannabis restores abilities and health, artists and scientists who use cannabis to enhance creativity, and meditators and ritual magicians who have incorporated the plant into their practices. I think it's important for us to share this kind of information about how we can use cannabis safely, effectively, and in our best interests.

As prohibition recedes, science advances. In some ways, this book is even more difficult to write now—our knowledge of the plant, including genetics, evolution, history, and pharmacology, grows faster than a hemp field in summer.

I waited many years to write this book, for the political and societal signs to shift a bit. The origin of this book goes back about twenty years to the Starwood Festival, which was then held at a site in rural Western New York state. That year, Stephen Gaskin, founder of The Farm community and author of *Cannabis Spirituality* (High Times, 1998), presented a workshop in which he discussed cannabis in relation to Eastern philosophy. The presentation inspired (after some discussion with Stephen) my own cannabis workshop the next year, focusing more on magick and the Western esoteric tradition. That turned into a long-running series of classes and generated a lot of useful, exciting, and stony information and techniques. Much of that—and more—will be found in the coming pages.

When I say that I am working on a book about cannabis and magick, the first question I get is "Why cannabis?" This question, I think, is largely motivated by a lack of knowledge of the eons-long history of cannabis use in magick and meditation and by belief in some of the myths and fallacies used by prohibitionists. The short answer is that cannabis can (with the proper techniques) help to induce a state in which the processes and results of magick become more probable and effective. The longer answer, which addresses both "why" and "how," will be found in the coming pages. Read on.

Is cannabis magick for everyone? Probably not. But the historical record and the scientific evidence strongly suggest that it can be an important adjunct for many. And as decriminalization spreads worldwide, the confluence of magick, yoga, meditation, and cannabis will become more and more common. In the past, information about this plant was purely occult, hidden away from law enforcement and disapproving eyes, and now we have the opportunity—and the responsibility—to shed new light on this misunderstood corner of esoteric spirituality.

CANNABIS
BASICS

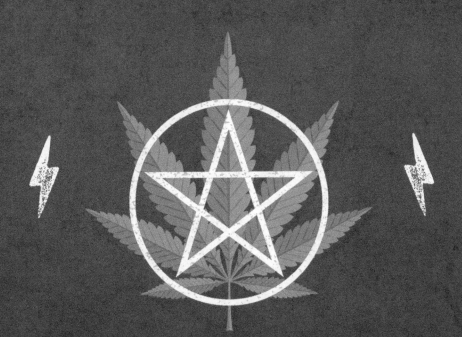

CHAPTER ONE
THE USEFUL PLANT

To the sadhu in meditation, cannabis is a gift from the god Shiva. To the Rastafari, it is the tool that helps people reason with each other. In popular culture, though, cannabis is the butt of snide jokes, an intoxicant that turns intelligent people into gentle idiots. Or maybe it is an evil "gateway" to harder drugs. At best it is a recreational intoxicant or an alternative medicine. As Aleister Crowley once wrote, "Comparable to the Alf Laylah wa Laylah itself, a very Tower of Babel, partaking alike of truth both gross and subtle inextricably interwoven with the most fantastic fable, is our view of the Herb—Hashish—the Herb Dangerous."[1] So, exactly what is cannabis?

The cannabis plant is a hardy, leafy-green shrub that has followed humans and evolved with us for thousands of years. As soil warms in the spring, cannabis seeds sprout and reach for the sun. The young plants spread dark green, wide leaves, grow for a season, mature, go to seed, and die back, although in more fortunate warmer climates, plants may survive and grow year-round. The plant has two sexes: male plants that produce little ball-like staminate flowers and females that produce clusters of tiny green flower bracts with white, hair-like pistils. These clusters are popularly called buds.

Every part of the plant is useful, and throughout history, cultures have discovered and rediscovered the numerous uses of cannabis. The roots are a

---

1. Crowley, Aleister. "The Psychology of Hashish." *The Equinox*, vol. I, no. 2, September, 1909.

source of medicine and can also be used to enrich the soil of other crops; the stalks are a source of fiber for rope, paper, and textiles; the seeds are a nutritious source of food and oil; the leaves are also a source of medicine as well as recreational beverages and biomass for distilling fuel; and the female flowers are medicinal and magical, the source of ganja and hashish.

There is some debate whether the varieties of cannabis should be classified as one species, as three, or even as four individual species. The most current genetic research suggests that all the psychoactive strains are *Cannabis indica* (divided into "narrow leaf drug" (NLD) varieties and "broad leaf drug" (BLD) varieties). Plants categorized as actual *Cannabis sativa*, the new thinking goes, are nonpsychoactive fiber hemp, but commercial NLD cannabis is generally referred to as "sativa," and we'll stick with the traditional varietal names here.[2] Whatever taxonomic classification the academics might eventually decide upon, we generally recognize three different varieties: sativa, indica, and Ruderalis. What we refer to as sativa varieties (actually NLD *Cannabis indica*) are typically tall, airy plants. These are quite potent and renowned for an uplifting, spiritual, psychedelic kind of high, excellent for magical and meditative uses. Indica (BLD) plants are usually squat, dense, resin-rich plants with a more relaxing "body" high. Ruderalis, also called "autoflowering" or "dwarf cannabis," is a tiny variety that distinguishes itself not only by being very short, but also by flowering whenever and wherever it pleases, regardless of season or the length of day. In ancient times, Ruderalis strains were a source of medicine and psychoactive cannabis but were long forgotten. Recently they have experienced a comeback among cannabis growers. We generally refer to the plants used for fiber or seed as "hemp" and the ones grown for medicine, magick, and fun as "ganja" or "marijuana," though they are really all the same plant: *Cannabis*.

With the exception of Ruderalis, cannabis plants rely on the length of daylight to let them know what kind of growth to produce. When days are long in summer, the plants concentrate on "vegetative growth," growing branches and leaves. When days become short in the fall, the plants shift into flowering, the males producing pollen and the females producing buds and seeds. Some

2. Clarke, Robert C., and Mark Merlin. *Cannabis: Evolution and Ethnobotany*. University of California Press, 2013.

cannabis strains are acclimated to a short northern growing season, while others can only be grown outdoors in the tropics. Indoor cannabis growers mimic natural light cycles using timers to stimulate growth and buds at the appropriate times.

This hardy weed grows pretty much everywhere on planet Earth, with the possible exception of Antarctica. While it sometimes escapes and does well on its own, almost all known varieties are cultivars, plants grown and bred by humans for human purposes. Numerous diverse strains have been developed. In China and other places, plants grown for food produce clusters of enormous, oversized seeds. In places where hemp is grown, fiber plants are tall with a single thick stalk. In Central Asia (and many other places), plants grown to make hashish are dense little Christmas trees. In Thailand, where the plants can grow year-round, big, bud-laden sativas resemble oaks or maples, growing twenty or thirty feet tall. In many parts of the world, indoor plants are bred to grow well in modern hydroponic systems with artificial light. Outdoor medical plants in California yield huge quantities of bud on gigantic single-season bushes. Wherever you are, there's a cannabis variety that will somehow, some way, grow there.

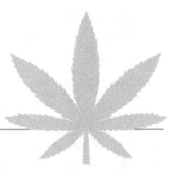

CHAPTER TWO

FORMS AND USES

Most cannabis users in Western culture are familiar with only one aspect of cannabis use: smoking the stuff. That's an important aspect, of course. But it is far from the only way we can approach this useful plant. Understanding the many ways to use the different parts of the plant can provide a basis for magical and spiritual applications. Think of these methods as you might instructions in other fundamental ritual techniques, such as drawing a circle, finding qabalistic correspondences, or using divination.

ROOTS

The roots of the cannabis plant contain amino acids and steroids, among other medicinal chemicals. We find the roots used in folk medicine throughout the world to treat inflammation, headaches, difficult childbirth, and as a health tonic. In general, they are prepared by soaking dried roots in either water or alcohol to create medicinal decoctions.

Cannabis roots also hold onto nitrogen and plant nutrients that other crops may leach from soil. Planting cannabis between other crops and tilling the roots back into the ground can replenish soil and restore depleted farmland.

STALKS

Stalks are sometimes also used in creating medicines, but more often they are used to create fiber for rope and textiles. In a process called retting, the stalks are soaked in water until the fibers begin to separate. The fibers are then cleaned of any excess organic matter and woven into twine, rope, or fabric. Fabrics made from cannabis are very strong and durable. Canvas was originally made from hemp (and the word "canvas" itself is a corruption of "cannabis"), as was denim. That's right! The original American blue jeans were weed!

Sometimes the rope, fabric, or raw stalks are used for symbolic or magical purposes. Stalks may be used as magical wands. Impressions of hemp cord pressed into pottery may have had a ceremonial meaning in ancient China and other places. Hemp fabrics are used not only for durable, everyday garments, but also for dedicated ritual robes and other ceremonial clothing.

LEAVES

For a long time, growers in the US would harvest their plants, save the buds for drying, and throw away big piles of leaves. Only recently has the value of the leaves been rediscovered. Raw, fresh leaves contain large amounts of medicinal chemicals. Fresh cannabis is usually not psychoactive the way that dried ganja can be. It can act as a mild stimulant, and has antibiotic, anti-inflammatory, and possibly even anticancer properties. A daily fresh cannabis drink can be a wonderful health practice.

In India, the fresh leaves are made into a beverage called *bhang*, which is sacred to the god Shiva and served to all at festivals in his honor. Bhang is said to confer joy and long life and is used as a sacramental drink. There are at least several forms of bhang, made variously from fresh leaves, dried leaves, or fresh or dried flower tops. Here's a traditional fresh-leaf method:

Recipe for Fresh-Leaf Bhang[3]

Soak 50 grams of fresh cannabis leaves in warm water for 5 minutes, then drain. Avoid rinsing the leaves under running water, as this may wash away the resin glands from the surface of the leaf. Chop the leaves as finely as you can, then mix with melon seeds, cucumber seeds, and black pepper. Add ½ liter of water and ½ liter of milk and then sweeten to taste with sugar or honey. Put it

---

3. Ratsch, Christian. *Marijuana Medicine: A World Tour of the Healing and Visionary Powers of Cannabis.* Healing Arts, 2001.

in the blender for several minutes or, if you want to be more traditional, churn and mash everything together with a stone, a pestle, or a garlic hammer until well blended.

A modern version of fresh-leaf bhang can be made by running fresh leaves through a vegetable juicer. About one tablespoon of pure cannabis juice makes a single dose. For taste, this can be combined with fresh carrot juice or any other kind of juice. Since most of us may have very limited access to fresh leaves, when they come around they can be juiced and the juice frozen for later use. An ice cube tray can be used to freeze individual doses. The cubes can later be thawed and added to milk or other beverages. Remember, this only works with the fresh stuff, right off the plant. A bag of dried herb that you bought for smoking will not make juice.

Now here's something interesting: if you take fresh juice—or bhang produced by either recipe—and heat it, it will lose some of its medicinal value—but it will become psychoactive. Sometimes very psychoactive. Remember that the juice may be very concentrated, and when heat converts the chemicals into THC, there may be a lot of it. If you experiment in this way, drink cautiously until you know the potency!

Some people also eat the fresh leaves whole, like salad, as a way to gently clean the digestive tract. I would suggest that if you do this, keep it to just a leaf or two at a time and avoid the leaf stems. Larger quantities of whole leaf cannabis (not juiced) can be a stomach irritant.

FLOWERS

When you go into an Amsterdam coffeeshop or a marijuana dispensary in the US, Canada, or Uruguay, what you will mostly find are dried cannabis flowers. These are the buds that herb smokers are familiar with, the resin-rich tops of the female plants. When the flowers are harvested, the leaves are trimmed away and the buds are slowly dried. This converts some of the chemicals in the plant into psychoactive cannabinoids, most notably THC and CBD.

Buds from different types of cannabis can vary widely in potency, quality of the high, taste, and smell. Poorly stored commercial cannabis, cannabis from nondrug strains, or weed that has been improperly grown and harvested can have very little active effect and you might need to smoke a whole lot before you feel anything. Excellent, well-treated, top-quality bud can be very, very potent and may require only a small amount to get you very, very high.

SMOKING AND VAPORIZING

Most people smoke the buds in joints, pipes, or bongs. In Europe, for many years, smokers mixed their cannabis with tobacco, which I do not recommend. Tobacco is addictive and can cause cancer and the combination with cannabis may be even more unhealthy than tobacco alone. If you are going to smoke, keep cannabis pure.

We'll talk about the health aspects of smoking later, but for now suffice it to say that studies show that smoking pure cannabis has few, if any, health consequences.[4] But if you remain concerned about the amounts of tar and combustion byproducts in your smoke, then stick with joints, which are often more efficient than pipes, water pipes, or bongs.[5]

If you don't like smoke for whatever reason, you can vaporize your ganja. Vaporizers are devices that heat the cannabis to the point where the resin evaporates, but the plant material does not burn. This produces a light, white vapor that retains more of the flavor of the buds and little or no tar and combustion products. There are several types of vaporizer on the market today, many quite good. The least efficient ones use a glass globe to catch the vapor. Some of the better varieties draw hot air through a glass wand or ceramic chamber, producing a thick vapor hit like the smoke from a bong (but not smoke at all). Some use forced air to fill a plastic bag or balloon with vapor that can be passed around. The newest trend in vaporizers are handheld "vape pens" that can produce vapor from dried herb or cannabis extracts of various kinds.

Whether you are smoking or vaporizing, the method is simple. You inhale deeply and hold it in for three to five seconds. During that time, up to 90 percent of the active chemicals are absorbed by your lungs. Some people like to

---

4. Tashkin, Donald P. "Effects of Marijuana Smoking on the Lung," *Annals of the American Thoracic Society.* Vol. 10, no. 3, June, 2013.

5. Gieringer, Dale. "Marijuana Water Pipe and Vaporizer Study," *Newsletter of the Multidisciplinary Association for Psychedelic Studies.* Vol. 6, no. 3, Summer, 1996.

hold their smoke in longer, but there is no evidence that it gets you any higher.[6] In fact, there is some evidence that only minimal holding is necessary.[7]

Smoking or vaporizing is, generally, a very efficient method for getting cannabis into your bloodstream. It also allows you to titrate your dose. That is, an experienced cannabis user can smoke until he or she reaches the desired level of psychoactivity and can then set the joint down.

Popular lore holds that modern cannabis is more potent than weed of the past. It's not really true, but even if it were, good! The stronger the better, because when we titrate doses, we might only need to take a single toke or two. That further cuts down the amounts of tar and combustion products that we might inhale while giving the same effect as an entire joint of lesser ganja.

COOKING WITH CANNABIS

Many people like to cook with their dried buds. In Amsterdam, everyone loves the space cake. In the US, pot brownies have long been popular and a wide variety of cannabis edibles are available in the states where it is legal. In Thailand, Nepal, and other parts of the world, cannabis buds are considered a culinary herb and may be a common ingredient in curries and soups, lending a distinct flavor and a mild buzz. When properly prepared, cooked cannabis can be a pleasant and effective way to ingest the stuff. However, it is not nearly as efficient as smoking. The cannabis must pass through the digestive system and takes a very long time to absorb. It may be as long as two full hours before you feel even the slightest tingle from your space cake. This can lead to the second problem with eating cannabis: it is very difficult to titrate. I've seen it happen too many times—someone eats a brownie, waits an hour, and decides they aren't getting the effect they want, so they eat another. And so on, consuming way more than they can comfortably handle before it even kicks in![8]

6. Holland, Julie (ed.). *The Pot Book: A Complete Guide to Cannabis*. Park Street Press, 2010.

7. Rabinski, G. "Surprise: Most of us have been inhaling cannabis the wrong way," Green Flower Media, 2016. https://www.green-flower.com/articles/95/best-way-to-inhale-cannabis-2016-3.

8. Dowd, Maureen. "Don't Harsh Our Mellow, Dude," *The New York Times*, June 3, 2014. https://www.nytimes.com/2014/06/04/opinion/dowd-dont-harsh-our-mellow-dude.html.

At the worst, of course, those brownie munchers became delirious for a while and fell asleep. They were fine the next day. But you do need to exercise some caution and know how potent your cookies are before you start in on seconds. Unfortunately, since potency of dried bud can vary quite a bit, it is impossible to give recipes that produce the same strength brownies for everyone. You'll have to experiment a little to find the recipes and dosages that work for you. If you are fortunate enough to live someplace where the THC content of edibles is listed on the label, aim for about ten milligrams of THC in a dose, and then titrate up or down from there on subsequent experiences.

The active ingredients in dried cannabis are fat soluble but not water soluble. That means that you'll need some kind of oil or fat in your recipe and the buds will need to be gently heated with the oil to make them orally active. The simplest way to do this is with the Leary biscuit (named after Tim Leary, who was fond of this method).

Leary Biscuit

Take a cracker and place a small- to medium-size bud on top. Spray with cooking oil or coconut oil. Microwave for a short time, until you see the resin start to run into the oil (it will turn green or brownish). Eat.

Mostly, cannabis chefs will dissolve the plant resin in butter or oil, strain away the crunchy bits, and use the fat as you normally would in a pastry recipe.

Green Butter

Take a ½ ounce of dried bud or trim and grind thoroughly. In a small saucepan, add the ground herb, ½ pound of butter, and ½ cup of water. Melt the butter and bring to a gentle boil. Simmer for 3 hours with the lid on. The butter should now be green. Pour through a fine screen or cheesecloth and then pour a small amount of boiling water through the solids that remain in your filter, washing any remaining butter from the herbal material. Save the strained liquid and dispose of the herbal solids. Pour the liquid into a bowl and refrigerate, undisturbed, overnight. The next morning, you will find that the butter and water have separated, leaving a solid chunk of green butter floating on top of the water. Using a fork or spatula, carefully lift the butter from the water.

Dispose of the water and sediment and use the green butter in your favorite pastry recipe. This also works well with coconut oil or any other fat that will turn solid when refrigerated.

KIF, HASHISH, AND OTHER CONCENTRATES

Good buds sparkle with what appear to be little crystals of cannabis resin. In reality, these aren't crystals but resin-producing glands called trichomes. When the trichomes are separated from the rest of the plant material, this concentrated form of resin is known as kif. When the kif is warmed and pressed into a solid form, we usually call that hashish or charas.

In some cultures, the resin is collected by hand-rubbing the tops of live plants. The sticky trichomes are then scraped from the skin and rolled into balls of charas. While this isn't a very efficient method to gather resin, it does produce hash of exceptional, indeed legendary, quality. Some aficionados believe that resin collected from living plants is more potent and more enjoyable than resin collected from harvested and dried herb.

More commonly, the kif is collected by shaking or rubbing dried buds over a piece of silk or fine screen. The trichomes fall through the screen, where they can be collected. Some cannabis enthusiasts will use a kif box to prepare their buds for smoking. The kif box or pollen box has a silk screen for a bottom and collection tray beneath it. By using it as a surface to crush buds and roll joints, a little bit of resin falls through the screen every time. After finishing a bag of weed, the enthusiast can then pull out the collection tray and be rewarded with a bowl or two of kif. Bonus!

A modern method of kif collection uses ice water to freeze the buds, causing the trichomes to fall off, through a filter bag. This is called water hash or bag hash.

Smoking kif or hashish is much like smoking bud, only more potent. Some of the subtlety of flavor of the buds may be lost, but charas has its own characteristic taste and smell, which some smokers find preferable. Again, experienced smokers will titrate doses and will not get any higher than someone smoking bud—they will simply use less. As with bud, potency and quality can vary greatly. In Europe, a common type of cheap hashish called "soap bar" may be adulterated with any number of ingredients that, if you knew about them, you wouldn't want to smoke or ingest—and it doesn't get you very high. At the more magical end of the hashish range, temple balls from Nepal are very potent, very high-quality, hand-rubbed charas that have been dedicated to Shiva and intended for ritual use.[9]

In recent years, other kinds of cannabis concentrates have become popular, including hash oil, which isn't really hash but a concentrated extract of plant resins and oils. Active ingredients may be extracted using a variety of solvents, including olive oil, alcohol, benzene, naphtha, butane, and CO_2. Finished products range from a green, sticky goo, to a substance that looks like amber wax and is often called honey oil or wax. When well-extracted, this may preserve much of the subtlety and flavor of the whole buds.

There are pros, cons, and obvious dangers and health issues that come with each of these extraction methods. Olive oil extracts an excellent range of cannabinoids and terpenes, but once dissolved in the oil, they stay there; it can't be concentrated any further. Olive oil extracts are a good edible or topical form of cannabinoids and cannot be smoked or vaporized. Extraction with ethyl alcohol is fairly safe and the finished product can be concentrated or left in a little bit of alcohol as a tincture. Alcohol-extracted oil can be very potent and easy to smoke or vaporize, but the alcohol captures too wide a range of chemicals and it may contain a lot more than just cannabinoids and terpenes, giving it an unpleasantly "green" taste and a sticky consistency. Naphtha and benzene are very efficient solvents but are also toxic chemicals that are unhealthy to be around. Even a miniscule amount of benzene residue in your oil could be carcinogenic. Butane extraction is very efficient and produces a very high quality and, if properly prepared, safe-to-use end product; the downside is that the extraction process itself is very dangerous. (Also, it should be noted, butane is a petroleum by-product and use of it supports an out-of-control fossil fuel industry and contributes to global climate change.) The growing popularity of "butane honey oil" (also called dab, wax, or shatter) has led to increasing numbers of headlines about gas explosions. CO_2 extraction is a much safer way of

---

9. Matthews, Patrick. *Cannabis Culture*. Bloomsbury, 2000.

producing honey oil; however the equipment necessary is uncommon and expensive, more suitable for a professional pharmaceutical company.

Hash oil is usually consumed either by vaporizing it in special pipes, "dab rigs," and vape pens designed for the purpose or by ingesting it orally. It can also be used topically.

GLYCERIN EXTRACTS AND E-JUICE

Cannabis resins can also be extracted in vegetable glycerin or food-grade propylene glycol. These extracts can be used sublingually—a few drops under the tongue will get you high quickly and without the fuss or odor of smoking. They also make a superb topical ointment. Glycerin extracts are also used in e-cigarettes and vape pens and are sometimes referred to as "e-juice." (Commercial e-juice may also contain propylene glycol and other less desirable chemicals, so caveat emptor. In 2019, news headlines began to describe a vaping-related lung illness that affected thousands and was responsible for over thirty deaths. This was due to blackmarket e-juice products, not from vaporizing dry herb, pure hash oil, or wax. To be on the safe side, use glycerin extracts topically or orally and do not inhale!)

Making a Glycerin Extract

Pulverize 5 grams of high-quality bud. Place in a mason jar with 40 ml of food-grade vegetable glycerin (make sure it says "food grade" or "kosher" on the label), which will probably be just enough to saturate the herb. Sit the jar in a pan of water and simmer gently for 2½ hours. Remove from heat and place in a safe, dark place. Let the jar sit for 2 weeks, shaking it vigorously once a day. Then scoop out the contents into a piece of cheesecloth. Squeeze the glycerin out into a cup and, when you think you've gotten every last drop that you can, dispose of the cheesecloth and spent ganja. The glycerin should now be a brownish or golden color and will smell like fine hashish when rubbed on the nose.

CBD OIL/ISOLATE

CBD products have become extremely popular and widely available in spite of being illegal at the federal level. That's right: as of this writing, even though marketers continue to claim that CBD is legal in all fifty states, it has never been de-scheduled and remains a Schedule 1 drug in the US. Marketers argue that since it is mostly manufactured from THC-free industrial hemp, it is as legal as other hemp products, including seeds and seed oil. It isn't, but that hasn't stopped anyone, apparently.

CBD is mostly used for medical and not magical purposes—it has enormous potential as an anti-inflammatory, antiseizure, and antipsychotic agent. It has quite a few medical uses and very low psychoactivity. However, it is way more effective when combined with even small amounts of THC and probably also interacts in a positive way with terpenes and flavinoids.

There are a few drawbacks, though. One is that CBD may affect how other drugs are metabolized. If your medication has a "grapefruit warning" on it, that also applies to CBD, which can affect the same biochemical pathways as grapefruit. Another drawback is that, being illegally produced, quality control may be less than you might hope for. Industrial hemp is not regulated for use as food or as a drug and growers often employ pesticides and chemical fertilizers that may become concentrated in an extract.

If you want to explore CBD products for medical use, I recommend finding a source that uses high-CBD strains grown as they would grow high-THC strains. That is, get it from a dispensary or a grower and be wary of the stuff you find in smoke shops and convenience stores.

STORAGE

Well-stored cannabis can last up to a couple of years before it starts to lose potency. The worst enemy of cannabis molecules is light; cannabis in any form should be kept in the dark. The resin tends to bond with plastic after a while, so keeping it in a plastic bag or other plastic container should only be used as a short-term solution. Glass, particularly dark brown or green glass, is the best way to go. Excessive heat will also destroy your weed, so keep it cool. Sealed containers of properly dried weed can be kept in the refrigerator—but not in the freezer; any small amount of water left in the herb will freeze, expand, and break down your buds. While some smokers like to keep their ganja a little bit moist, drier bud will actually last longer. If you are using a vaporizer, drier herb will vaporize more easily, too, though it may taste harsher in a pipe or joint. Ideally, finished bud should be thoroughly dry yet still fairly pliable and sticky with resin. To sum up: keep your weed dry, cool, and in a dark place!

FREQUENCY OF USE

The mantra that you've probably heard repeated any number of times concerning cannabis: everybody is a little bit different and everyone responds with slight—or not so slight—differences. In general, though, the less frequently you use cannabis, the stronger your response; the more often you use it, the more tolerance you will develop. Daily users may be able to smoke very strong herb and not bat an eye, while someone with less tolerance than Willie Nelson may find themselves very, very stoned. With that said, some people respond very positively to full immersion and daily use, while others will need to experiment much less frequently and pick strategic times and places. A basic rule of Psychoactives 101 comes into play for almost everyone—wait until your work (as well as driving, using power tools, etc.) is completed before you get high.

If you do use cannabis regularly, taking a break of a few days to a few weeks will help to reset your receptor sites and will lower your tolerance, allowing smaller amounts to go much further.

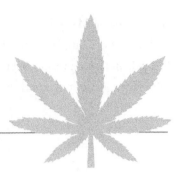

CHAPTER THREE

THE SYMBOL
OF THE LEAF

The shape of the cannabis leaf is one of the most identifiable leaf-shapes on the planet, known to probably billions of people who couldn't pick an oak leaf out of a lineup of maples. Depictions of cannabis leaves appear in archaeological findings dating back many thousands of years and from every part of the civilized globe. In our culture, the leaf can be seen everywhere, adorning clothing, album covers, product packaging, books, magazines, and more.

The cannabis plant provides us with its own symbolism that works on a variety of levels. As with the experience of cannabis itself, the more you explore, the more you reveal. The leaf, as I'm sure you know, is composed of an odd number of leaflets—usually five, seven, or nine, but sometimes more or less depending on the genetics and age of the individual plant—radiating out from a central point at the end of the leaf stem. The configuration suggests a grouping of united elements. Like all good symbolism, it can have multiple interpretations:

The Plant of Many Uses: The cannabis plant is a unique ethnobotanical that has, historically, been used for medicines, incense, textiles, rope, food, oil, fuel, and much more. Every part of the plant is useful in some way, each use being a leaflet that is united by the common ancestry of cannabis.

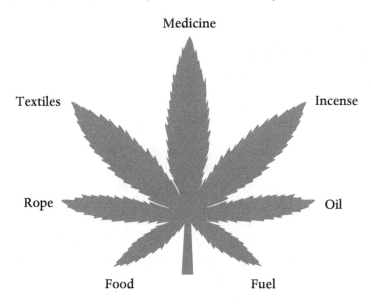

The Entourage Effect: The medicinal, cognitive, and spiritual uses of cannabis depend on a variety of chemicals in the plant working together. Over one hundred cannabinoid chemicals have been isolated and each has its own effects and modifying actions on other cannabinoids. In addition to the cannabinoids, there are also terpenes and flavinoids, again each having its own effects and modifying abilities. Like a set of leaflets of varying sizes joining together, the cannabinoids, terpenes, and flavinoids of an individual plant join together to produce the overall effect of the plant.

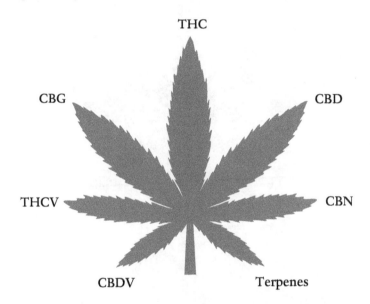

Ritual Community: Cannabis has an affinity for naturally generated ritual. In many situations, the ritual of getting high will organize participants into a circle, each person like a leaflet radiating from the common center, the cannabis itself.

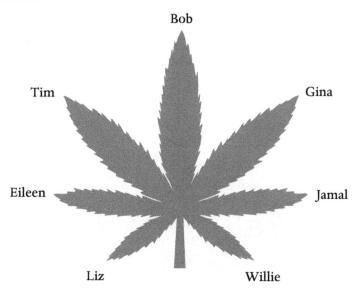

Reality Selection: At every moment, our minds make choices about what we like, what we believe, what we experience, and how we represent and express our likes, beliefs, and experiences to ourselves and to others. Smoking or ingesting psychoactive cannabinoids allows some of this process to move from preconscious into conscious awareness. Each of those choices, from the meanings applied to language to the ways that we process basic sensory perceptions, helps to define our reality, the overall experience of the world in which we live. Cannabis allows us to choose with a more conscious awareness of what we are doing, to select our experience. When we make these choices, each option can stand revealed, a collection of leaflets united and culminating in a decision.

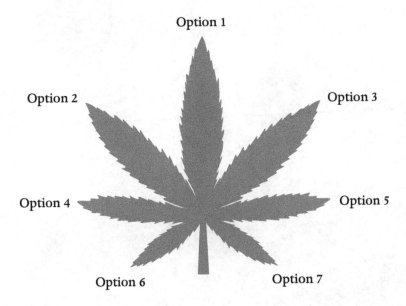

Each of these leaves will be explored further in the pages ahead.

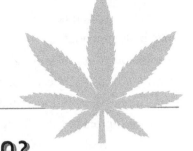

CHAPTER FOUR
TOWARD A CANNABIS QABALA?

Occult qabala is a system of categorizing the contents of human experience, both the world itself and the internal consciousness of the individual. Based in the older system of Jewish mysticism, usually known as Kabbalah, qabala makes use of a diagram known as the Tree of Life to divvy up reality into ten "spheres" (Sephiroth) and "paths." Quite a bit of magick tradition is based on qabala, including many tarot decks, and several systems of creating ritual. Almost any field of knowledge may be usefully categorized on the Tree of Life, with common charts, found in numerous books on magick, listing the correspondences for deities, ranks of angels, tarot cards, plants, animals, minerals, perfumes, and just about everything else. Long-term practice of occult qabala can result in a better understanding of the processes of mind, a sense of how the elements of life are interconnected, and the ability to quickly create rituals. Eventually, when we are able to categorize strains of cannabis and cannabinoids on the Tree of Life, it may facilitate the creation of cannabis rituals and allow the magician to choose which strains or chemicals are useful in which situations. Unfortunately, that may be some years away, as the cannabis plant, in all its variety, may be complicated to categorize.

The plant contains a range of active ingredients, mostly cannabinoids and terpenoids, only a few of which are well studied. Our bodies produce their own counterparts to the cannabinoids found in the plant, interesting chemicals including anandamide, noladin ether, 2-AG, and others, that stimulate or moderate body functions.[10] These chemicals act on at least two types of receptors that are found in cells throughout the brain and body, denoted CB1 and CB2. In general, the CB1 receptors are found in the brain and nervous system and the CB2 receptors are found in the immune system and organs. Small amounts of CB1 receptors are also found in the body and some CB2 receptors are also found in the brain. This system of receptors has become increasingly important to medical science; it appears that the endocannabinoid system works as a master switchboard for metabolism, mood, hunger, motivation, immune, and many other functions. So it seems like a fortuitous coincidence—or clever foresight and breeding by our distant ancestors—that an easily cultivated plant should hold so many keys to our wellness and consciousness.[11]

All of this information about cannabinoids, receptor sites, and so on is very recent. The human endocannabinoid system was not even dreamed of until the 1970s and was barely understood until the twenty-first century. Careful observers of consciousness, though, were figuring it out centuries ago, or at least one century ago in Aleister Crowley's case. His 1909 essay "The Psychology of Hashish," while bumping hard against the limits of science of the time, makes some uncannily accurate observations and also gives some broad hints concerning the magical applications of cannabis.

Crowley described what he believed were three separate actions of cannabis upon his mind and body: the volatile aromatic effect, the toxic hallucinative effect, and the narcotic effect. The volatile aromatic effect he characterized as a state of "perfect introspection" in which "one perceives one's thoughts and nothing but one's thoughts, and it is as thoughts that one perceives them." The toxic hallucinative effect he described as a higher dose experience in which "the images of thought pass more rapidly through the brain, at last vertiginously fast. They are no longer recognized as thoughts, but imagined as exterior."

10. Bisogno, T., Ligresti, A., and Di Marzo, V. "The endocannabinoid signalling system: biochemical aspects." *Pharmacology, Biochemistry, and Behavior 81,* June, 2015.

11. Pacher, P., Batkai, S., and Kunos, G. "The Endocannabinoid System as an Emerging Target of Pharmacotherapy." *Pharmacol Rev. 58,* 2006.

And finally, the narcotic effect, he told us, produced sleepiness. Crowley theorized that the three effects were the result of three separate substances in the plant material. He also noted that different samples he encountered seemed to have varying amounts of these substances and that one sample produced only the sedative effect.

We now know that there are dozens of active chemicals in cannabis, with varying excitatory, hallucinatory, calming, or other qualities. Our modern concept of plant cannabinoid activity is increasingly based on what researchers call the entourage effect. In short, cannabinoids and terpenoids work better—and differently—in combination with each other and different combinations yield different medicines and different experiences.[12] Crowley may have had an inkling about the entourage effect and was very much on target in his observations that cannabis acts through multiple chemicals and that different samples have different effects. Beyond that, he was hinting that hashish was a Eucharist, something to be consumed as the substance of deity. Specifically he was demonstrating that cannabis was a "Eucharist of three elements" that conformed to the three gunas, the universal tendencies described in Hindu philosophy: sattvas, rajas, and tamas. Sattvas is the tendency toward balance, purity, and lucidity. Rajas is the tendency toward activity, movement, or change. Tamas is the tendency toward inactivity, darkness, and lethargy.[13]

While these tendencies are certainly found in the effects of cannabis, there's no simple division into three active chemicals, as Crowley may have imagined. There are dozens of cannabinoids found in different proportions in plants from different genetic lineages, different growing techniques, and different geographical locations. Six of them are perhaps somewhat better studied than the others and when cannabis samples are tested for medicinal use, the amounts of each of the six are often determined. These are THC (delta-9-tetrahydrocannabinol), CBD (cannabidiol), CBN (cannabinol), CBG (cannabigerol), THCV (tetrahydrocannabivarin), and CBDV (cannabidivarin). In general, plants grown for psychoactivity typically have more THC than anything, but

12. Russo, Ethan B. "Taming THC: Potential Cannabis Synergy and Phytocannabinoid-Terpenoid Entourage Effects." *British Journal of Pharmacology*, 2011, 163 1344–1364.

13. Crowley, Aleister. *Magick in Theory and Practice*. Dover Publications, 1976.

also other cannabinoids in small but significant proportions. Plants grown for fiber or seed often have more CBD than anything else, but again, they still have other cannabinoids in small but significant amounts. There are exceptions to this rule—indeed, as the medicinal properties of CBD become more widely known, high-CBD strains are becoming more popular among patients and tokers. Occultists reading this may be working out some of the permutations of the six chemicals already. Each combination of cannabinoids creates unique mental and physical effects. How many unique cannabinoid profiles might be useful, fun, or magical?

But wait! Cannabinoids aren't all you get in cannabis. Like other herbs consumed by humans, the cannabis plant is rich in aromatic chemicals called terpenoids. These are the same sweet, spicy, sour, fruity, and flowery substances that give herbs, teas, pines, fruits, flowers, and many others their tastes and smells. And, as any herbalist can tell us, they have medicinal and psychoactive properties of their own, some of which parallel those of the cannabinoids. One of the most common terpenoids in many strains of cannabis is beta-caryophyllene, also found in cinnamon, black pepper, and other spices. Beta-caryophyllene is unique among the terpenoids studied so far in that it also seems to act in a small way on the CB2 cannabinoid receptors. Other common terpenoids in cannabis include alpha-pinene (also found in pine trees), beta-myrcene (found in hops, myrrh, and others), limonene (lemon), linalool (lavender), and nerolidol (orange), among many others. The combination of terpenoids gives each strain of cannabis its unique aroma and taste. Again, each terpenoid has its own medicinal and/or psychoactive effects and each of them combines with other terpenoids to create unique effects. The evidence is very strong, too, that the terpenoids are active participants in the entourage effect with the cannabinoids.[14]

So the cannabinoid/terpenoid profile of a strain of cannabis, or even each individual plant, is as unique as the crystal structure of a snowflake. For instance, one breeder reports that at one harvest their strain of White Widow contained a large amount of pinene, a smaller amount of trans-caryophyllene, and only a trace amount of a few other terpenoids along with high levels of

---

14. Russo, 2011.

THC and much smaller amounts of CBD and CBN. Alternatively, their strain of El Nino sports even higher amounts of THC, lower amounts of CBD and CBN, and a large quantity of myrcene as the dominant terpenoid followed by smaller quantities of pinene and other terpenoids. Of those two strains, White Widow is often rated as the stronger one even though the El Nino actually has more THC.[15] Both have unique taste, smell, and effect, and an experienced toker might be able to identify the strain from its aroma, flavor, or high.

So it's all a bit more complicated than the three mystical constituents that Crowley theorized. If we wanted to attribute cannabinoids and terpenoids to the gunas, we might relate the brain-arousing, paranoia-inducing, hallucinogenic THC to rajas, along with the stimulating THCV and, perhaps, beta-caryophyllene. The antianxiety, brain-calming cannabinoid CBD might be a candidate for tamas, along with sedative terpenoids like myrcene or nerolidol. I submit that Crowley's perfect cannabis experience of sattvas clarity might be induced more by a balanced combination of cannabinoids and terpenoids rather than by any single one of them. Indeed, in experiments in which subjects were injected with either pure THC, pure CBD, or a balanced combination of the two, most subjects disliked the pure THC, were unimpressed by the pure CBD, and rated the combination as effective and pleasant.[16]

While we didn't even know cannabinoids existed until recently, terpenoids and magical practice have crossed paths many times. Any number of occultists have outlined or studied the qabalistic correspondences of essential oils, herbs, and other terpene-rich substances. A complete qabalistic accounting of cannabis would need to develop correspondences for both individual cannabinoids and various entourage combinations of cannabinoids and terpenoids. Attributions might be developed based on comparisons to plants with similar terpenoid profiles, from the medicinal properties of the dominant constituents and from evaluation of the subjective experience. As cannabinoid testing of

15. "Strains Terpenes Analysis." Green House Seeds, Netherlands. http://www.greenhouse seeds.nl/shop/strains-terpenes-profiles.html.

16. Brunt et al. "Therapeutic Satisfaction and Subjective Effects of Different Strains of Pharmaceutical-Grade Cannabis." *J Clin Psychopharmacol* 2014; *34: 344 Y 349*); see also: Intravenous THC and cannabidiol Experiment. https://www.youtube.com/watch?v=T2cAFRAX3Gs.

plant material is a very recent trend, it may be some years yet before magicians have enough practical experience of samples with known profiles to create a useful cannabis qabala.

Until then, some occultists have simplified the process by mixing their cannabis with other magical herbs. If you have a particular herb that you work with *and it is smoke-able or edible*, then you can mix small amounts into the cannabis that you smoke, eat, or vaporize. In general, magicians will look up the qabalistic, astrological, or other attribution of an herb in one of the many resources available online or in books.[17]

---

17. One classic would be Crowley's volume *777*, which lists qabalistic correspondences for herbs, stones, perfumes, deities, and more.

CHAPTER FIVE

MAGICAL HISTORY

The real history of cannabis is often a little difficult for modern minds, indoctrinated in antidrug hysteria, to wrap around. Wherever the magical plant was available, spiritual traditions evolved around it; shamans, priests, and worshipers used cannabis in divination, consecration, prophecy, ritual, and meditation. Some even contend that it was influential in the birth of human spirituality itself. That's a sweeping and powerful statement—with compelling, if little-known, evidence. Of course, given the prevailing prejudice against the plant, these are controversial ideas, and short of time travel, there's no way to confirm anything absolutely. At the very least, based on the written and archaeological record, we can say with certitude that human spirituality coevolved with entheogens, psychoactive plants that activate the mystical parts of our brains, and that cannabis was one of the more frequently used ones.

Cannabis was certainly one of the first cultivated plants, and by the time recorded history rolled around, it was being used for fiber, food, medicine, recreation, and ritual.[18] Some have even suggested that it was *the* first cultivated plant.[19] Remember that no other plant is as useful as cannabis. It is the only plant that with a little help from humans produces almost everything needed

---

18. Schultes et al. *Plants of the Gods: Their Sacred, Healing, and Hallucinogenic Powers.* Healing Arts Press, 2001.

19. Sagan, Carl. *The Dragons of Eden: Speculations on the Evolution of Human Intelligence.* Ballantine Books, 2012.

to build a civilization. To the ancient people who really needed to build a civilization, it must have seemed particularly magical.

And so the earliest references that we find are glowing and reverent. A legendary Chinese figure, the Red Emperor, Shennong, is said to have compiled the first pharmacopoeia in 2737 BC, giving an honored place to cannabis. Not only did he recommend it medicinally for a variety of ailments but also as the principle ingredient in an elixir of immortality. The elixir had the power to transform a mortal into a transcendent being. Cannabis, he claimed, enabled seekers to forget their own consciousness and attain the Tao.[20]

Cannabis remained a medical necessity in China for hundreds if not thousands of years. With the advent of Confucianism, magical and spiritual use waned. However, Confucianism's alternative, Taoism, continued and even deepened its relationship with the plant. The more mystical and alchemical side of Taoism embraced the use of cannabis in incense and potions of various kinds. The ancient Taoists celebrated eight major deities, or immortals, and one of them was Ma Gu, which is usually translated as "Hemp Maid" or "Auntie Hemp." She embodied the spirit of the cannabis plant and presided over the slopes of Tai Shan mountain in the hemp-producing region of Shandong. Pilgrims would travel to Tai Shan mountain and toss hemp seed from the heights, a ritual action intended to bring health and longevity. Some of the many legends about Ma Gu may be based on actual women whose exploits were rolled into one syncretic deity.[21]

Ma Gu is always represented as an eighteen-year-old woman, although her real age is infinite. She is known as Immortal Xu Miao, Infinite Harmony.[22] In Vietnam, images of Ma Gu adorn restaurant plates to this day, accompanied by the saying "Ma Gu Xian Shou," which translates as "Hemp Maid Offers Longevity."[23]

20. Ratsch, 2001.

21. Clarke and Merlin, 2013.

22. "Who is Ma Gu?" Way of Infinite Harmony, 2019. https://www.wayofinfiniteharmony.org/who-is-magu/.

23. Clarke and Merlin, 2013.

Just over the mountains in Central Asia, a collection of tribes known as the Indo-Europeans had a new invention, the wheeled chariot pulled by horses, and they were in the process of spreading their culture all over the place. Between 4000 and 1000 BC, the Indo-Europeans, sometimes called Aryans, migrated into India, Mesopotamia, and a big part of what would become Europe. The central ritual of their culture, which they carried wherever they went, involved a sacrament known as sauma or soma.[24] The soma ritual took root everyplace the highly mobile Indo-Europeans visited.

In the 1960s, an ethnomycologist and banker named R. Gordon Wasson published a beautiful, deeply researched volume that suggested that soma was a mushroom, *Amanita muscaria*. The book traced the history of soma in the ancient texts of the *Rig Veda* in early Hindu lore and the related haoma in the Avesta of the Zoroastrian tradition and helped to promulgate the idea that an entheogen may have been at the root of religious traditions. Alas, as later ethnobotanists pointed out, and archaeological evidence confirmed, soma was probably not a mushroom. It may have been a number of plants over time, as the original "moon plant" of the *Rig Veda* was, much later, banned, lost, confused, etc. But the description of the plant, having leaves and branches and extracted by mixing with milk, just as bhang is still made today, fits cannabis more so than any other herb. This is especially the case when we start to examine the spiritual properties of soma, the "elixir of immortality" and "bringer of laughter," as well as haoma, which is described as a sweet-scented, golden-hued plant that grows in the mountains, can assume the shape of a cane, tree, or bush, and can produce food, medicine, and rope.[25] That seems to be a very specific description of cannabis.

Indeed, a soma/haoma "factory" or temple of sorts was discovered in an archaeological dig in what was once the kingdom of Bactria, in the part of Central Asia (present day Turkmenistan, Afghanistan, Uzbekistan, and Tajikistan, north of the Hindu Kush mountains) where cannabis is thought to have originated. Dating from around 2000 BC, containers in the temple yielded the

---

24. Bennett, Chris. *Cannabis and the Soma Solution*. Trine Day, 2010.

25. E.C.D.Q. "Haoma's Identifying Features," The Church of Cognizance, 2006. http://dan mary.org/tiki/tiki-read_article.php?articleId=2.

ancient residue of several different plant combinations that included the ephedra herb, a stimulant, and the opium poppy. However, every combination had as its base—you guessed it—cannabis.[26]

In the Vedas, the language describing soma is beautiful:

Flow soma, in a most sweet and exhilarating stream, effused for Indra to drink. The all-beholding destroyer of Rakshasas has stepped upon his gold-smitten birthplace, united with the wooden cask. Be the lavish giver of wealth, most bounteous, the destroyer of enemies; bestow on us the riches of the affluent. Come with food to the sacrifice of the mighty gods, and bring us strength and sustenance. To thee we come, O dropping (soma); for thee only is this our worship day by day, our prayers are to thee, none other.[27]

In the *Rig Veda*, soma was associated with Indra, a mighty warrior who was king of the gods. Indra was a thunder god who took great delight in drinking soma. In addition to his never-ending battle against demons and other opponents of the gods, he is one of the guardians of the directions, ruling the east. Interestingly, he is described as having the yellow hair and Caucasian features of an Indo-European and it seems likely that Indra (and, probably, Shiva) were brought to India by the Aryans.[28]

Indra also appears in the Avesta, drinking haoma, though he does not have the same importance he has in the Vedas. In the Avesta, a number of deities appear, with more importance given to the haoma-quaffing Mithra. We'll get back to Mithra in a little bit, but what do you say we check in with the Indo-Europeans?

If we go back to calling the Indo-Europeans "Aryans," it's easier to remember that they were tall, blond, Caucasian people. So when we find the remains of shamans in various places, with blond hair and stashes of cannabis buried with them, we might think that the Indo-Europeans spread their canna-

---

26. Bennett, 2010.

27. *Rig Veda, 9th mandala.*

28. Anthony, David W. *The Horse, the Wheel, and Language: How Bronze-Age Riders from the Eurasian Steppes Shaped the Modern World.* Princeton University Press, 2007.

bis spirituality far and wide. One recent finding of a Caucasian mummy, over twenty-seven thousand years old and found in the Gobi Desert, yielded nearly two pounds of cannabis tops in good enough condition to see that it was once primo herb. And the shaman's gear buried along with the mummy suggests that the ancient ganja was for healing or spiritual purposes.[29]

One of the heirs to Aryan traditions was a wide-ranging nomadic people known to us as the Scythians. Also proficient with horses, around 600 BC these warrior-shamans swept out from their Central Asian homelands and conquered a vast swath of Europe, Asia, and the Middle East. Along with their horsemanship and prowess in battle, the Scythians were known for wearing tall, conical hats, sometimes covered with mystical symbols, and they were frequently covered in tattoos. Their culture was based heavily on the use of cannabis for food, fiber, medicine, and religion. The Scythians had no written language but left behind a variety of intricately created art objects that tell stories through pictograms. Their principal deity was Tabiti, a goddess of fire, cannabis, and horses, not surprisingly. The Scythians were known by a variety of names in the languages of the people they encountered, including the Saka, the Ashkenazi, and the Haomavarga or "haoma-gatherers." In turn, their word for their favorite herb was *kannabis*, which comes down to us today almost unchanged.

In 450 BC, the Greek writer Herodotus described a Scythian funeral rite in which mourners gathered in a small tent. A bronze cauldron was filled with cannabis and heated. The tent would fill with cannabis vapor and the participants would cry out in ecstasy. Archaeological finds have confirmed the use of cauldron-vaporizers, some of them weighing up to seventy-five pounds and still containing residue of Scythian ganja.

Among the Scythian warriors were the enaries, shamans and magicians who used cannabis to induce trance and prophesy. The enaries were mostly men who dressed in women's clothing and uttered their pronouncements

29. Viegas, Jennifer. "World's Oldest Marijuana Stash Totally Busted," *Discovery News*, December 3, 2008. http://www.nbcnews.com/id/28034925/ns/technology_and_science-science/t/worlds-oldest-marijuana-stash-totally-busted/.

in high-pitched voices. The cross-dressing symbolized crossing between the earthly world and the world of spirit.

Also found in the remains of ancient Scythian camps were devices for inhaling smoke on a more personal basis. These did not seem to be connected to a particular ritual and it is theorized that they were for recreational use.[30]

Throughout the range of the Scythian empire, we find all three types of cannabis and it is suspected that they used the sativas for fiber and food, the indica for medicine, and the Ruderalis for spiritual and recreational purposes. The Scythians spread cannabis and its use throughout the then-known world. When they began to settle down, the Scythians merged with the indigenous populations in the Middle East, India, Europe, and the British Islands.[31]

Elements of cannabis culture and ritual passed from the Scythians to, among many others, the Thracians. The nomadic Thracians became known for their ability to produce fine hemp cloth. They also continued the Scythian tradition of weed smoke prophecy. Much of the prophetic fun was associated with their deity, Dionysus, who was a Thracian pothead before he became a Greek wino. Among the Thracians, the shamans who danced and used cannabis to enter ecstatic trance were known as *kapnobatai*, "those who walk in smoke."[32]

The list of cultures influenced by the Scythians is lengthy, representing most of the inhabitants from the Celtic islands to India. For our purposes, an important Scythian connection would be with the ancient Semites. The Scythians rode into Judea around 625 BC and thereafter had a long history fighting beside and trading with the people of Judea and surrounding nations. The Bible records the use of an herb called *kaneh-bosem*, which, in days gone by, was translated as "sweet cane" and thought to be the calamus plant, a marsh grass that yields a fragrant, but not easily psychoactive, essential oil. Several historians have argued that kaneh-bosem was, instead, an Aramaic adoption of the

---

30. Bennett, 2010.

31. Ratsch, 2001.

32. Bennett, 2010.

Scythian word "kannabis," which does a better job of explaining the apparently entheogenic qualities of the holy anointing oil made from it.[33]

In the book of Exodus, it is forbidden to anoint anyone other than priests with the oil and priests who had been anointed were forbidden to leave the temple while high. Anything that the oil touched would become sacred and the anointing rite was later used to consecrate the Hebrew kings, who were literally drenched in the stuff. In Exodus, there is an account of Moses burning the oil as incense in an enclosed temple-tent to get some advice from his deity, a practice very similar to the rituals of the Scythians.[34] The Torah refers to the pillar of smoke that arose from Moses's incense as the *Shekinah*.

Meanwhile, back in Persia, Zoroaster returned from a trip to the haoma temple in Bactria (the same one later excavated by archaeologists) with revelations about a new religion based around the haoma rite.[35] The Zoroastrians celebrated their haoma rite in praise of Mithra, and with Zoroaster's new revelations fresh in hand, things started to change. While some historians maintain that Zoroaster prohibited the use of haoma, the rite persisted and, in fact, is still practiced by Zoroastrians today. Verses in the Avesta show that Zoroaster spoke in praise of haoma but against *mada*, an intoxicant that some writers have associated with haoma but may have been a very different drug altogether.[36] Over time, it seems that the original psychoactive ingredient was removed from the sacrament, perhaps an attempt to reserve direct mystical experience for a priest caste, or to differentiate Zoroastrianism from the surrounding indigenous shamanic traditions. The rite is still practiced today, but the haoma is made from ephedra or Syrian rue, without the cannabis and without the mystical depth described in the ancient texts. The word "magi" was originally the term applied to the caste of priestly Avestans into which Zoroaster was born, and who probably kept the original, psychoactive haoma ritual for themselves

33. Benet, Sula. "Early Diffusion and Folk Uses of Hemp." *Cannabis and Culture*, Rubin, Vera & Comitas, Lambros (eds.). De Gruyter Mouton, 1975.

34. Russo, 2011. Bennett, 2010.

35. Bennett, 2010.

36. Eliade, Mircea. *A History of Religious Ideas, Vol. 1.* University of Chicago Press, 1978.

long after it was prohibited for lay Zoroastrians.[37] In a sense, at least etymologically, cannabis may have been at the very origins of what we now call magick.

Scholars largely agree that Christianity incorporated quite a bit of mythology and practice from Zoroastrianism, with many parallels to be noted between Mithra and Jesus Christ. I'll leave that for a class on comparative religion, but I can highlight some of the juicy, ganja-related bits. Initiates into the cult of Mithra would be taken through a seven-step process, each step likely being an experience derived from a plant drug, including, of course, the haoma. The seven sacraments of Mithra worshippers remain in their modern form as the seven sacraments of the Roman Catholic church, which still include among them the Eucharist and the anointing oil. Jesus himself is described in the New Testament as using the anointing oil to heal and cast out demons. Indeed, the name "Christ" itself comes from *chrism*, anointing oil, and means "the anointed one."[38]

At the Last Supper, Jesus lifts the sacraments and offers up soma. While this is usually taken as the Greek word for "body," it seems odd that J. C., who was speaking Aramaic in the early texts, would insert a Greek word. If the Eucharistic cup contained a psychoactive ingredient, as a number of historians have suggested, then Jesus was making a pun, intentional or not. The modern Catholic Mass may easily be considered as a carryover or a reflection of the original soma/haoma sacrament, with placebos replacing the historically more potent "body of the god."[39]

Back in India, oceans of bhang were still being poured as offerings and consumed in honor of the gods, but the deities were shifting around. Indra, fond of his soma, was falling out of favor and Shiva, another pre-Hindu deity who may have originated with the Indo-Europeans or the Scythians, was gaining favor. Shiva, the lord of yoga, among many other titles, gained a seminal place in every version of the Hindu creation myth. Some scholars have even argued that Shiva is really a continuation or slight alteration of Indra with the names changed to protect the very, very high.

---

37. *Oxford English Dictionary*. Bennett, 2010.

38. *Random House Unabridged Dictionary*, Random House, Inc., 2019.

39. Bennett, 2010.

Another change that happened along with the shift in deities is that soma became forbidden except for use by the priests. Oddly, bhang remained in common use. What was the difference? Apparently a ritual was needed to transform the cannabis infused milk into the sacred beverage.[40] We likely see the vestiges of the soma transubstantiation in the Roman Catholic mass, in which a ritual transforms wine and crackers into the flesh and blood of the god.

Amrita was the elixir of immortality of the gods, a vast ocean of milk that needed to be pressed and churned, just as a bowl of soma might be prepared, only on a godly scale, creating the world itself. The churning was dangerous. The amrita was poisoned and it fell to Shiva, and a snake, to purify the milky ocean. And it was messy. When the sacred nectar spattered from the heavens, wherever a drop landed, a cannabis plant would grow. Shiva found the plants and gave them to humans so they might experience delight, courage, and heightened sexual pleasure. Shiva is also the master of yoga and with his guidance the yogi might achieve good health, long life, and visions of the gods through the use of ganja. Even today, dreadlocked sadhus consecrate their smoke to Shiva as a meditation practice and bowls of bhang are churned and purified in Shiva's honor.[41]

Again, nearly everywhere cannabis traveled on planet Earth, it was adopted for spiritual, meditation, or magical use. When it made its way into Africa, it was immediately welcomed by the local shamans. Medicinal, spiritual, and recreational use is documented throughout the continent. In Zambezi, tribal ceremonies are similar to those of the Scythians with participants inhaling vapors from cannabis heated upon an altar. The Kasai tribes of the Congo treat the cannabis spirit as a deity who protects against physical and spiritual harm. The Kasai also use cannabis ritually, smoking to seal deals and treaties. The use of cannabis both ritually and recreationally goes back centuries among the Hottentots, Bushmen, and Kaffirs.[42] Among the Twa in Rwanda, cannabis is said to

---

40. Ibid.

41. Schultes, 2001.

42. Ibid.

make a connection to the ancestors—who also used cannabis incense in their rituals.[43]

In the Arabic world, cannabis has a long association with the mystical Sufi traditions. While Islamic doctrine specifically forbids the use of alcohol, some sects adopted hashish as a tool to enter states of religious ecstasy and meditative wonder. Some Sufi dervishes, much like the Shiva sadhus, would renounce worldly possessions, live by begging, and smoke copious quantities of hashish while praying and meditating.

The moniker "The Green One" was applied by Sufis to both cannabis and a saint who embodied the spirit of the plant, al-Khidr or Khizr. In some traditions, Khidr was an alternative name for the prophet Elijah and in others he seems a version of the dying and resurrected vegetation deities that we find in many mythologies. He is dismembered and then not only restored but made immortal by the water of life. Getting high was referred to as "a visit from Khidr." It is likely that the Khidr legends predate Islam altogether and may be a carryover from Avestan/Zoroastrian traditions that once flourished in the same part of the world.[44]

Many of these traditions still survive in a variety of forms. In Morocco, the Joujouka tribes, who lived isolated in a mountainous region for hundreds of years, claim descent from an early Sufi group. Their tradition of smoking kif all night while playing music, dancing, and invoking their deity, Boujeloud, harks back to ecstatic Sufi prayer methods, though it seems to have fused with local Pagan mythology.[45]

When we examine the historical evidence honestly, it really does seem that a shared fiber in the origins of many world religions was the magick herb cannabis.

---

43. Ratsch, 2001.

44. Bennett, 2010.

45. Woodruff Leary, Rosemary. "The Master Musicians" in Paul Krassner (ed.), *Psychedelic Trips for the Mind*, reprinted 2000; Leary, Timothy. *Jail Notes*. New York, 1971.

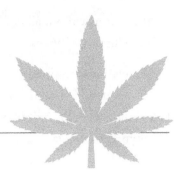

CHAPTER SIX

MORE RECENT HISTORY

Through the Middle Ages and the Inquisition, cannabis use in Europe as part of the magick and ritual of many non-Christian traditions became a secretive activity. As such, most of the references we find are in a kind of code. In the 1500s, the monk Francois Rabelais wrote a series of exceptional satires titled *Gargantua and Pantagruel*. In one memorable chapter, Rabelais describes how the characters stock a ship for a sea voyage; the principle item to be stocked, used for just about everything, is the "Herb Pantagruelion," which is certainly cannabis, named after one of the tale's heroes, Pantagruel.

> It is likewise call'd Pantagruelion, because of the notable and singular Qualities, Virtues and Properties thereof: For as Pantagruel hath been the Idea, Pattern, Prototype and Exemplary of all Jovial Perfection and Accomplishment, (in the truth whereof, I believe there is none of you, Gentlemen Drinkers, that putteth any question) so in this Pantagruelion have I found so much Efficacy and Energy, so much Compleatness and Excellency, so much Exquisiteness and Rareity, and so many admirable Effects and Operations of a transcendent Nature, that if the Worth and Virtue thereof had been known, when those Trees, by the Relation of the Prophet, made Election of a Wooden King to rule and govern over

them, it it without all doubt would have carried away from all the rest the Plurality of Votes and Suffrages.[46]

Rabelais was an important influence on two later literary figures pertinent to our discussion. The first was Shakespeare, who borrowed happily from Rabelais's literary style and subject matter. The Bard may also have emulated the monk in another way; pipes with cannabis residue were found at the site of Shakespeare's home in Stratford-on-Avon, dating from the time when he lived there and wrote his plays and sonnets. Shakespeare may also be making a Pantagruelian allusion when he writes about "a noted weed" in Sonnet 76:

Why is my verse so barren of new pride?
So far from variation or quick change?
Why with the time do I not glance aside
To new-found methods and to compounds strange?
Why write I still all one, ever the same,
And keep invention in a noted weed,
That every word doth almost tell my name,
Showing their birth, and where they did proceed? ...

For some clarification, "weed," as the Bard uses it here is a pun. In the slang of the time, "weeds" referred to clothing, and the clothing of the day was mostly hemp. So he is comparing literary style to clothing, while suggesting a further property of hemp, "invention." [47]

The other author influenced by Rabelais was the twentieth-century occultist Aleister Crowley, whom we shall discuss in more depth later.

There is evidence that cannabis was employed by medieval and Renaissance alchemists for a variety of purposes, including the quest for the philosopher's stone. While some alchemists pursued a physical stone that would serve as universal medicine, elixir of immortality, and transmuter of metals, others took the language as symbolic of an inner, personal transformation. Some of these

46. Rabelais, Francois. *The Works of Mr. Francis Rabelais: Doctor in pysick, containing five books of the lives, heroick deeds & sayings of Gargantua and his sonne Pantagruel*, translated by Sir Thomas Urquhart, Peter Anthony Motteux, G. Richard, 1904.

47. Bennett, Chris. *Liber 420*. Trine Day, 2018.

most likely used our favorite plant, along with other psychoactive substances, though the language remains symbolic and obtuse to hide the practice from the uninitiated. Even worse, long associated with shamanism, Pagan rites, pre-Christian religions, and various Islamic sects, cannabis use, if discovered, was a shortcut to the inquisitor's torture chamber. As a result, a "green language" was developed, in which the names of other plants and objects were substituted for the more controversial herb. A common code for cannabis in alchemy was the "green lion."

Some were a little more obvious. In 1604, alchemist Heinrich Khunrath published a treatise entitled *Amphitheater of Eternal Wisdom*. Among several engravings in the volume is one titled "The First Stage of the Great Work," featuring an alchemist kneeling before the opening of a very Scythian-looking tent. Beside the alchemist is a fuming censer, with the words "ascending smoke, sacrificial speech acceptable to God" written in the billowing cloud. Khunrath also described the special transformative ingredient that he used as a "red resin," an adequate description of the red Lebanese hashish that would have been available to him at the time.[48]

Along with the creation of the philosopher's stone, the physical alchemists were adept at making spagyric extracts of herbs. The process is essentially the same as modern extraction techniques to produce hash oil (a tincture that may or may not contain the aromatic essential oil, depending on the methods used) with the added step of burning the extracted plant material and introducing some of the ash to the oil. This was to make sure that the extract held everything that was in the whole plant, making spagyric extracts even more whole than the whole plant and broad spectrum extracts offered for sale in medical dispensaries. I can't say whether or not this increases the medical or spiritual nature of the extract, but it can be thought of as a reiteration of the holistic theme represented by the leaf symbol.

---

48. Bennett, Chris, Lynn Osburn, and Judy Osburn. *Green Gold the Tree of Life: Marijuana in Magic and Religion*. Access Unltd, 1995.

P. B. RANDOLPH

Paschal Beverly Randolph was a nineteenth-century doctor, magician, and Rosicrucian. Randolph, an African American, was a friend of Abraham Lincoln, an early campaigner for civil rights, and the largest importer of hashish into the US. He studied with the mesmerists in Europe and traveled to Egypt, where he first encountered hashish and became fascinated with the magical potential of the herb.

Randolph's pioneering work with sex magick—and his use of cannabis—was a big influence on many later occultists, including Aleister Crowley.[49]

ALEISTER CROWLEY

Crowley is probably the best-known, or at least most infamous, practitioner of magick in the twentieth century. A world traveler, chess champion, mountain climber, magician, and writer, the depth and volume of his occult explorations have rarely been equaled by anyone. He founded at least one magical order and was the head of at least one more. His legend was confounded by the yellow press of his day, which held him to be a Satanist and "the wickedest man on earth," the first being false, and the second having many more evil contenders (Crowley, it seems, could be pretty obnoxious, borrowed money from everyone, and loved to puncture the taboos of others, but he was not a criminal, murderer, or "black magician," as the stories purported). He was also, apparently, an agent of British intelligence who worked to get America into World War I.

Crowley experimented widely with cannabis, opium, mescaline, ether, and other drugs, mostly for their occult properties. Cannabis and mescaline were apparently his favorite magical catalysts and he wrote about them in symbolic, veiled terms.[50]

---

49. Bennett, Chris. "The Hidden Hash Master of the 19th Century: Paschal Beverly Randolph," Cannabis Culture, November 12, 2016. https://www.cannabisculture.com /content/2016/11/12/hidden-hash-master-19th-century-paschal-beverly-randolph/.

50. Kaczynski, Richard. *Perdurabo: The Life of Aleister Crowley.* New Falcon, 2002; Sutin, Lawrence. *Do What Thou Wilt: A Life of Aleister Crowley.* St. Martin's Griffin, 2002.

RASTAFARI

The Rastafari are spiritual and magical cannabis users known to the world through the words, deeds, and songs of reggae musicians such as Bob Marley and Peter Tosh. While there are organized forms of Rastafari religion, such as the Twelve Tribes or the Nyabinghi, most Rastas consider it a way of life rather than a religion and encourage each practitioner to seek within for their own truth.

Rastafari began in Jamaica in the 1930s as a messianic tradition that considered Emperor Haile Selassie I of Ethiopia an incarnation of Jah, the God of the Judeo-Christian bible. Cannabis is an important part of Rasta ritual, meditation, and daily life. Some consider the practice a reclaiming of African tradition and there is also a strong influence of both Hindu and Sufi tradition. Like the sadhus in meditation, Rastas grow their hair in long dreadlocks and make liberal use of a chillum, a traditional pipe for smoking ganja, called a "chalice." As with both sadhus and Sufi dervishes, the use of cannabis is more of an ascetic practice, part of a turning away from the mass culture of "Babylon," rather than a sensual one.

Rastas use the herb that they call "the healing of the nation" to gain insight from Jah. They consider cannabis a sacrament given to humans to heal and cleanse body and mind, exalt consciousness, and come closer to their deity. A smoke is shared when Rastas come together to "reason" or meditate together. A reverent attitude is usually expected and someone unable to be calm and peaceful may be ejected. In the past, smoking ganja as a spiritual practice was reserved for men. Women, alternatively, used and prepared edible cannabis for medicinal purposes. That seems to be changing, with women now claiming a greater role in all aspects of Rasta life.

> [Cannabis] is important for a purpose and that purpose is different for all people. Like for me, me use my herb as a meditative kind of thing. When you meditate, when you read a Bible or you write songs, you use the herb because your mind is set in such a way that...there are more things...that you see. This is what herb is for. It's not something out of space or ridiculous. Herb is there for a purpose. It's for the mind and

the body, too, because we drink it or eat it. I'm a say that meditative purpose is important part of marijuana use. Relaxation of the mind. Focusing of the mind on your spirituality, on the Almighty. This is herb and this is the purpose of herb for some. —Ziggy Marley, musician and son of Bob Marley[51]

OTHER MODERN CANNABIS SECTS

As in every other historical epoch, where cannabis grows, spiritual and magical traditions arise. In our time, the illegality of the plant has kept these new religions small and persecuted, yet adherents persist even though they risk arrest or worse.

In 2006, the founders of the Church of Cognizance, Dan and Mary Quaintance, were arrested in Arizona with 172 pounds of cannabis. The Church of Cognizance holds that cannabis is the original haoma and that the sacrament is "the teacher, the protector, the provider" that inspires "good words, good thoughts, good deeds."[52]

Roger Christie, founder of THC Ministry in Hawaii, was arrested by federal agents in 2010 on possession and trafficking charges. THC Ministry believes in the use of cannabis for meditation, prayer, healing, fellowship, and formal rituals such as weddings and funerals.[53]

It is unfortunate that for many of us our spirituality must be inherently a revolutionary act, a rejection of cultural norms and attitudes. I prefer when a student sits to meditate or practice ritual that the meditation or ritual is the only thing he or she has in mind. Perhaps the day will come soon when this will be. In the meantime, we all must personally make the choice and decide how important we make our practice, whether it is worth the scorn and, indeed, punishment of our fellow citizens.

---

51. Interview with the author, 1993.

52. "Mission," Church of Cognizance. http://enlightener.net/coc/wiki/tiki-index .php?page=Mission.

53. Christie, Roger. "History, Beliefs, and Practices of the THC Ministry," THC Ministry: the Hawai'i Cannabis Ministry. http://www.thc-ministry.org/?page_id=362.

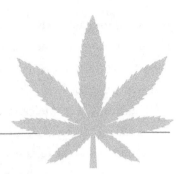

CHAPTER SEVEN

YOUR BRAIN (AND BODY) ON CANNABIS

Ancient civilizations that used cannabis placed a great deal of importance on the plant. They knew from experience what scientists have only recently discovered. While the existence of cannabinoid chemicals, the compounds that give cannabis its unique healing and psychoactive properties, was known as early as the 1940s, it wasn't until 1964 that Dr. Raphael Mechoulam isolated THC and identified it as the main psychoactive compound. And it wasn't until the 1980s that Mechoulam and his team identified the cannabinoid receptors in the human body and the "endocannabinoid system" (ECS), the set of receptors and internal chemicals that helps to maintain balance in quite a few organs and bodily systems.

The extent of the endocannabinoid system is still being revealed, but it has become obvious that it acts as a moderator, a control mechanism for a variety of immune, metabolic, and brain functions. Cannabinoid receptors are found not only in the brain but throughout the body with concentrations in the spinal cord and in the gut. There are two general types of cannabinoid receptor: CB1, which seems to be connected more with the "high," and CB2, which is connected more with somatic feelings and immune processes. There are subtypes of each, though the study of these is in its infancy. In general, the function of the ECS is to maintain balance, to inhibit or excite depending on what is needed in a particular system at a particular time. The endocannabinoid system maintains homeostasis, the delicate and ever-changing balance between the processes and systems of the human body.

The ubiquity of the cannabinoid receptors throughout the human organism—and the importance of maintaining homeostasis—helps to explain the broad effects and usefulness of cannabis as medicine. It can treat quite a few ailments because the endocannabinoid system is integral to so many physical processes. Think of the ECS as being akin to the endocrine system, nervous system or cardiovascular system in importance. "Cannabinoid medicine" will likely be a medical specialty of the near future. Indeed, at the moment, the internet and libraries are loaded with both clinical information about cannabis as medicine[54] and, even more, the media is inundated with anecdotal reports of seemingly miraculous cures of various kinds. We are more concerned with magick and spiritual use here, but there is certainly some crossover between magick and healing, and we'll explore those aspects when the time comes.

For now, let's take a look at what cannabis does in the human brain that might be applied to either magick or healing. Again, cannabinoid receptors are found throughout the brain with concentrations in the amygdala, cerebellum, and hippocampus.

LEARNING AND BRAIN CHANGE

It was once widely believed that, after it was formed in childhood, the brain would pretty much stay the same for the rest of its life, perhaps deteriorating slowly as we age or do unhealthy things. We now know that as we learn and experience, throughout our lives, the synaptic pathways and structure of the brain change constantly. This is known as plasticity and it appears that the CB1 receptors play a crucial role in how we learn. As neurons communicate with each other via bioelectrical signals and the release of neurotransmitters, they

---

54. International Association for Cannabinoid Medicines, https://www.cannabis-med.org/?l ng=en; Holland, 2010; Granny Storm Crow, "If the truth won't do, then something is wrong," Granny Storm Crow's List (of cannabis news and studies). https://grannystorm crowslist.wordpress.com/the-list/.

continually monitor themselves and each other. If a cell is signaling too much or too little or releasing too much or too little of a neurotransmitter, a nearby neuron will release endocannabinoids that either activate or inhibit the action at the synapse. As the connections between neurons are either strengthened or weakened by this process, old neural pathways are extinguished and new ones are formed.[55] This synaptic plasticity is controlled by the CB1 receptors, and if we are attempting to change our thought processes and ourselves via magick, this is a key process that must be accessed in the brain.

The same effects have been observed from plant-derived cannabinoids, which not only act directly on the receptors themselves but also stimulate the release of endocannabinoids at the synaptic level.[56]

EMOTIONAL MEMORY AND ORIENTATION

Large concentrations of cannabinoid receptors have been found in the amygdala, a pair of structures located on either side of the brain in the temporal lobe. The amygdala is important in processing emotional memory and in controlling memory reconsolidation. In these regions, the release of endocannabinoids appears to be the main mechanism by which emotional memories, both good and bad, are encoded or extinguished. The action of cannabinoids in these brain areas allows us to resolve and move past emotional trauma. Likewise, it may also help us to attach powerful, positive emotional states to other, more pleasant memories. Both of these processes may be useful in magick.[57]

There is also some indication that the amygdala is involved in creativity[58] and cannabinoids may stimulate that process.

---

55. Gerdman, Gregory L., and Jason B. Schechter. "The Endocannabinoid System." in Holland, Julie (ed.). *The Pot Book: A Complete Guide to Cannabis*. Park Street Press, 2010.

56. Ibid; Wolf et al. "Cannabinoid receptor CB1 mediates baseline and activity-induced survival of new neurons in adult hippocampal neurogenesis." *Cell Communication and Signaling*, 2010 8:12.

57. Gerdman and Schechter, 2010.

58. Asari et al. "Amygdalar Enlargement Associated with Unique Perception." *Cortex* 46 (1): 94–99, 2010.

Cannabinoid receptors also play an important role in brain areas responsible for orientation in space, including the hippocampus and the cerebellum.[59] This may account for some of the body feelings that we get when we're high, including sensations of lightness or floating.

WHAT WAS THE QUESTION?

The hippocampus is also the part of the brain that processes short-term memory. Experiences are processed in short-term memory before they are archived, as it were, in long-term memory. Cannabis is rather famous for disrupting short-term memory, and when very high, a cannabis user may lose their way in speaking full sentences, forget the most recent question asked them, or wonder just why they walked into the kitchen. While these are often humorous and sometimes annoying effects, they also may demonstrate how the cannabinoid system helps us to heal from trauma (by forgetting!) and how cannabis can help in magick and meditation: by keeping our minds in the present. Having a very short short-term memory helps to keep awareness in the moment of *now*.

THE DEFAULT MODE NETWORK

Human brains spend a hell of a lot of time sorting and searching. Every time we encounter a word, to some extent we have to sort through definitions and contexts and find the appropriate meaning. For example, the word "chair" can refer to many different kinds of seating equipment. In making sense of the word, our brains may flip through a few different kinds of chairs before fixing on the one that makes sense in the current context, perhaps the one that you're sitting in now. Usually this happens too fast for the conscious mind to track, but when we start to pay attention, we can notice the process.

Exercise #1:

Think of a time when you felt really, really good.

So what happened when you attempted to recall a time when you felt really good? Most people, when encountering a vague suggestion of this kind, will

---

59. Gerdman and Schechter, 2010.

find themselves recalling not just one, but at least several memories, and then comparing and contrasting for a few moments until finding one that comes closest to the criterion of "really, really good."

If this happened to you, what you just experienced was a process called *transderivational search*,[60] which is mediated by a feature of the human brain known to neuroscientists as the default mode network (DMN). Here's another example:

Exercise #2:
Picture a really sexy face.

Whose face did you end up picturing? How many faces did you have to look at and adjust before you settled on that one? How quickly did the process happen?

Okay, one more for now:

Exercise #3:
What's the most comfortable item of clothing that you own?

While the original concept of transderivational search was applied to linguistics, to the choices that we make in our words, these experiences of the DMN and sorting happen in every sense. We sort through images, voices, music, emotions, tactile feelings, and every other form of human perception and internal representation, with equal ease. And we do it, consciously or unconsciously, on and off through most of our lives.

The discovery of the DMN by neuroscientist Marcus Raichle was in part unexpected. Dr. Raichle was hoping to measure baseline activity in the brain, to provide a statistical basis to compare with experimental activities. The idea was that when it wasn't doing anything consciously directed, the brain would power down like the hard drive in your computer, a mental screen saver would come on and the brain scans would show, in general, less activity than when the subject was working a math problem or solving a jigsaw puzzle. When Raichle and his team placed subjects in the fMRI machine with no specific instructions

---

60. Dilts, Robert, and Judith DeLozier. *Encyclopedia of Systemic Neuro-Linguistic Programming and NLP New Coding.* Scotts Valley, CA: NLP University Press, 2000.

and scanned while they did "nothing," he found something odd. Certain areas of the brain, including the hippocampus, midline cortical structures, and some frontal cortex structures, would hook up in a new configuration and really go to work. Raichle didn't know what these brain areas were doing, chattering furiously to each other, but the brains were using 30 percent more energy than when the subjects were consciously working on mental activities.[61]

After years of study, scientists are figuring out what the DMN does. I'll cut to the short answer, so you can sort out what I'm getting at here.

The default mode network creates reality.

Or, to state it in a wordier but more accurate way, the DMN is a physical component of the human organism that mediates the largely nonmaterial process of delineating and experiencing our world. It is the engine of sorting in the brain that also mediates some of the important processes of magick. And understanding how the DMN works in the brain can give important clues as to how to create more effective magick. I promise that after you give yourself a moment to sort through the range of things your brain wants to include as "important clues" or "effective magick," I'll explain what I mean.

The DMN can be thought of as an engine of narrative. It starts with active experience in the hippocampus, where the brain processes short-term memory. This can be either something that you just experienced within the last, say, half a minute, or it could be something that you remembered, the memory being shunted back to short-term memory so that you can experience parts of it again. If it is a memory, it already comes with some notes in the margin from the last time it took a tour of the DMN. The notes in the margin come in the form of sensory markers called submodalities. These are the qualities that we use to fine-tune our perceptions, for instance, brightness, dimness, volume, size, distance, location, color, movement, shape, and so on. If the narrative created by the DMN—the story of your life—were a motion picture, the submodalities would be the lighting, camera angles, and sound design that are used to convey mood, passage of time, foreshadowing, and so on. Here's an example:

---

61. Marcus E. Raichle et al. "A Default Mode of Brain Function." *Proceedings of the National Academy of Sciences,* January 16, 2001, vol. 98, no. 2, 676–682.

Exercise #4:

Think of two things that are objectively the same (or pretty damn similar), but you like one and not the other. For instance, oak trees versus maple trees, Toyotas versus Hyundais, Coke versus Pepsi, pullover sweaters versus button-down sweaters, and so on. The stronger your feelings of like and dislike, the better.

First think of the thing you like and make a visual representation. Look at it in your mind. Eliminate context and background, so that you are only looking at the object in question. Notice where you have to aim your eyes to look at this imagining. Point to it. Notice the colors of the image—are they rich and vibrant or dull and subtle? Notice how large you have made the image, how far away from you it is, and whether the lighting in the image is bright or dim.

Now perform the same experiment for the thing you don't like. Notice the qualities of the representation you make. Eliminate context and background. Notice where you have to aim your eyes. Point to it. Are the colors rich and vibrant or dull and subtle? Notice how large you have made the image, how far away from you it is, whether the lighting in the image is bright or dim, if the focus is sharp or blurry, and if the image is moving or still.

Most people will notice some differences between these two internal representations. You will point to different locations or one will be larger, brighter, or more colorful than the other. Each one of us has a unique set of submodality tags that we apply, so the results of this experiment will be at least somewhat different for each person, but the lesson to be derived is that we represent images, sounds, feelings, tastes, and smells to ourselves with variations that let us know crucial information about the memories or imaginings. Often these submodality differences will be reflected in metaphoric language: something very clever might be "brilliant" (have a brighter internal representation); someone you feel uncomfortable with might be "distant"; a friend with a distinctive personality might be "colorful"; a dynamic person might be represented as "larger than life"; something you don't like "smells rotten"; and so on. In each case, the content of the memory remains fairly consistent, although some way of viewing, hearing, feeling, tasting, and smelling has been altered to convey a message. Those judgments and evaluations of perception help to adapt memories and experience into the greater narrative.

The default mode network, as the engine of narrative, is the seat of the imagination. It runs our fantasies, daydreams, visualizations, and hallucinations as tools to incorporate information into the overarching tale of our existence. The submodality choices carry emotional and evaluative information along with the tale. The way the choices are made, running through a super-position of multiple possibilities before collapsing to a single delineation, parallels the process of measurement and delineation of particles in quantum physics. In effect, each submodality nuance that our DMN attaches to a memory defines what kind of reality, what story, we inhabit. And the DMN makes those delineations quite frequently.

Except when it doesn't. For some reason, focused attention and DMN activity are mutually exclusive. This is why your third grade teacher told you to stop daydreaming—you can't solve an arithmetic problem while your DMN is operating. For that, you need focused attention from the prefrontal cortex, known as executive function. Normally, that kind of focused attention shuts down the DMN and, vice versa, your wandering mind can prevent focused attention.

Unless you're high.

One of many roles of cannabinoid chemicals in the brain is moderation of the default mode network. In brain scan studies, it was observed that smoked cannabis switches on the DMN—without fully deactivating the areas of the brain involved in executive function. Which means that when you are high, you can be focused and spacey at the same time, clever and creative, productive and imaginative.[62]

It means that your connection to the realm of imagination, myth, legend, symbol, and magical archetype can remain active while you engage in almost any activity. The most ancient texts that mention cannabis, some thousands of years old, tell us that the herb was used to communicate with the spirit realm. No matter how often it was repeated in Chinese medical texts, Indian sacred writings, African lore, Arabic traditions, and in writings from nearly every civilization that knew of the psychoactive qualities of cannabis, the whole "spirit realm" concept was usually branded primitive superstition and soundly ig-

62. Bossong et al. *Default Mode Network in the Effects of Δ9-Tetrahydrocannabinol (THC) on Human Executive Function*, PLoS One, July 31, 2013.

nored. But now we can understand that there is a real basis for the connection between the plant and the world of thoughtforms and imagination.

As well, what we can hold in focused attention is rather limited. In the 1950s, scientists determined that our conscious awareness can hold "seven plus or minus two" pieces of information at any one time.[63] However accurate that number might be, it certainly does seem that the DMN can work with quite a bit more information at any one time, including every derivation of a transderivational search, and every detail of a vast plot arc. This creates opportunity for mystical experience, for perceiving the connections and patterns between apparently disparate objects and ideas. At the extreme end of cannabis-influenced mystical experience, consider Aleister Crowley's 1906 "Vision of the Universal Peacock":

> The "millions of worlds" game—the peacock multiform with each "eye" of its fan a mirror of glory wherein also another peacock—everything thus. (Here consciousness has no longer any knowledge of normal impression. Each thought is itself visualized as a World Peacock...) 1:20 a.m. Head still buzzing: wrote above. Samadhi is Hashish, an ye will; but Hashish is not Samadhi...[64]

While Crowley apparently struggled, at that early date, with the role that cannabis might play in magick, his "World Peacock" is a fine description of a cannabis revelation, including the richness and depth of information in a cosmic-scale narrative and some interesting hints as to what submodality cues Uncle Al's brain might favor.

Let's return to the idea of transderivational search for a moment. Every perception induces some measure of sorting through a range of similar experiences, memories, emotions, and thoughts so that our brains can delineate and attempt to make some meaning. Cannabis takes this process that usually runs below the level of conscious awareness and brings it gently into ongoing

63. Miller, G. A. "The magical number seven, plus or minus two: Some limits on our capacity for processing information." *Psychological Review.* 63 (2): 81–97.

64. Crowley journal entry from OTO archive, quoted in L. Sutin, *Do What Thou Wilt.* St. Martin's Press, New York. 2000.

experience. That means that every moment blossoms with associations. Every thought spawns a thousand and everything you see, hear, and feel comes within a fractal, ever-changing entourage of similar images, sounds, and feelings.

Cannabis may disrupt short-term memory when you're high (experiential evidence of its action on the hippocampus, processor of short-term memory), but the flow of narrative creation continues unabated and you may find later that your experiences are written large upon on the screen of long-term memory. Ordinary events and objects become imbued with mythic importance. Your hand becomes the symbol of the universe's striving, a trip to White Castle becomes an epic quest, a sip of beverage becomes a peak experience, a visualized shape gains depth and form, music becomes even more moving and life-changing, and the elements of ritual exude their symbolic properties. And each perception becomes consolidated in memory with submodality markers denoting importance in the story of your life.

> [It] is the Quality of this Grass to quicken the Operation of Thought it may be a Thousandfold, and moreover to figure each Step in Images complex and overpowering in Beauty, so that one hath not Time wherein to conceive, much less to utter any Word for a Name of any one of them. Also, such was the Multiplicity... that the Memory holdeth no more any one of them, but only a certain Comprehension of the Method. [65]

Exercise #5:

Take a few tokes. Wait five to ten minutes for the effects to be felt. Then experiment again with the following:

1. Think of a time when you felt really, really good.

2. Picture a really sexy face.

3. What's the most comfortable item of clothing that you own?

Now perform the same experiment with some fresh questions:

65. Crowley, Aleister. *The Book of Thoth*. Samuel Weiser, Inc. York Beach, ME, 1974.

1. Think of a time when you felt as free as you ever have.

2. Picture your tallest friend.

3. What's the most exciting movie you've seen in recent years?

How were these experiences different than when you first attempted them, above (that is, assuming you weren't high when you experimented with them earlier)? What happened when you attempted this with new questions?

THE LETTERS GAME

This is a pretty simple game that makes use of some of the mental processes we've discussed here. It works nicely with two to four people (though it can be fun in a larger group, too, if you keep it moving rapidly). For the most fun, play a few rounds without cannabis, then get high and play a few more.

Pick a two or three letter combination, perhaps the initials of someone present. Then think of as many phrases as you can that begin with those letters. For instance, C. G. gives us crazy glue, clever girl, commanding general, code green, Cary Grant, etc. The funnier, the better. Take turns, or just shout them out when you think of them. Play for as long as you'd like.

Afterward, consider the game as an interplay between the brain's default network (making internal lists of words, picking them out, finding matches, etc.) and problem-solving focused awareness. How was it different to play not high and then high? Which took longer to find matching phrases? Which phrases were more interesting, clever, poetic, or funny?

CANNABIS PRACTICES

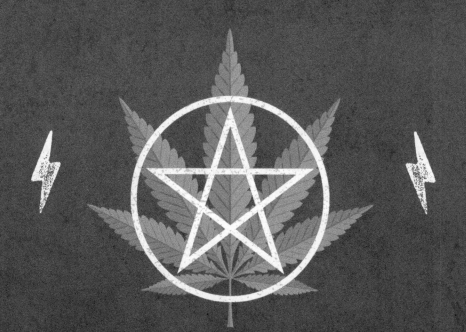

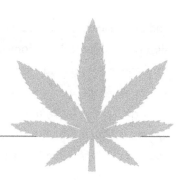

CHAPTER EIGHT
WHAT IS MAGICK, ANYWAY?

For some, magick is something that they do. For others, magick is something that they are. Some count only their spiritual or "nonmundane" behaviors as magick. Others consider only the paranormal or supernatural to count as magick. The broadest definition comes from Aleister Crowley, who defined his concept of magick as "the art and science of causing change in conformity with Will." While this is too inclusive for many practitioners, as it places almost every kind of human activity in the realm of magick, I rather like it. I like the idea that everything we do, from making breakfast to teaching to altering the very nature of reality itself, can be considered subject to the same intent and requirements. Crowley's definition encourages us to work to make every aspect of our lives, every moment, as magical as we can.

The key to Crowley's definition comes with the word *Thelema*, Greek for "will." The core teaching is "Do what thou wilt shall be the whole of the Law," a phrase that echoes Francois Rabelais's fictional Abbey of Thelema, where the only law was "Do what thou wilt." Crowley maintained that the first task of the magician was to find his or her true will, or natural purpose and direction through the universe. True will was understood through a process of ritual and appeal to the divine within. The "thou" in "Do what thou wilt," for Crowley, referred to the will of God or the universe rather than the wants, whims, and desires of the individual consciousness. So, in short, every action and decision can be magical if it conforms to the true, divine will.

Crowley, who studied chemistry while in college, considered science as a subset or a tool of magick and he encouraged its study.[66] His most secret magical order, the A∴A∴, used the motto "The method of science, the aim of religion." (Which fits with our scientific/magical exploration of cannabis, here and now.) His training in science may have been partly responsible for his keen observational abilities and, perhaps, his interest in entheogens. An experimental attitude and a healthy measure of scientific method allowed him to explore and develop ritual technologies in a way that the world had rarely seen before.

Crowley also suggested that, alongside science, mysticism was a part of a well-rounded magical practice. By mysticism he meant the practice of yoga and other forms of meditation designed to induce experiences of unity and wholeness, while developing concentration and control of the mind. The other, more directly magical branch of his system involves ritual.

Ritual is a fundamental human behavior. While we often think of it in the context of religion, we also create rituals—replicable processes that help to produce a desired state or result—in many other areas of our lives.

For instance, if you choose to have a romantic dinner with someone special, the ritual is simply to ensure that every aspect of the situation is aligned with the goal: the lights are dimmed, the candles lit, the champagne chilled, the food perfect, the music soft and suggestive. If you manage to arrange the circumstances for maximum woohoo, then an altered state is produced—a comfortable sharing, excitement, or erotic feelings—and your desired outcome of romance achieved. This ritual can be repeated with variations to achieve a romantic effect time after time.

Similarly, most of us have rituals that we use to prepare for a day of work, a night out with friends, a shower, or a sneeze. These are all delineated by space, time, behavior, and even state. The sneezing ritual might require fast hands and proximity to Kleenex; it might be over in just a moment, but it is a goal-directed ritual nonetheless, invoking qualities of health, safety, and cleanliness.

---

66. Crowley, 1976.

The sneeze itself is just a reflex action and doesn't quite rise to the level of ritual without the frame that is applied by covering the mouth, using a tissue, cleaning up, and perhaps saying thank you for the ritual "gesundheit" or "god bless you" offered by someone nearby. The frame aligns behaviors toward the goal. Each of these actions is elicited as a kind of anchored response. The first tickle in the nose and you look around for the tissue box, and so on. The ultimate outcome is the state of feeling well.[67]

The ritual frame influences everything that happens within it. Magicians have known this for eons, now science is reluctantly catching up. If you need that kind of reassurance, a double-blind study can be useful to confirm the obvious experience. In one recent study, participants were asked to perform either ritual actions or random gestures before consuming a snack. Chocolate, lemonade, and carrots were framed within rituals that involved unwrapping or other movements, compared with simply relaxing for a comparable amount of time or making random, nonritual movements. In the majority of subjects, the rituals increased their self-rated desire for and enjoyment of the snack, even the carrots, over the nonritual control snacks.[68]

Of course, our aims in magick are frequently greater and more interesting than how much we desire and like snacks! In general, we perform rituals for purposes of banishing, invocation, evocation, and making things happen. The banishing operations are usually for creating space in which to work and clearing away distractions and unwanted influences. Invocation is how we draw desired qualities and influences into our consciousness. Evocation is the art of communicating with entities external to us. And making things happen may or may not be the end result of all of this.

In many magical traditions, a systematic exploration of invocation and evocation is encouraged. That is, a magician draws in and contacts the qualities of the universe in a balanced and full way that leaves his or her consciousness richer, larger, more flexible and open, and perhaps a little wiser for it. The frameworks may involve holistic systems such as qabala, astrology, alchemy,

---

67. For more information, see my book *Brain Magick*.
68. Vohs et al. "Rituals Enchance Consumption." *Psychol Sci*, 2013.

Goetia, or the pantheons of any number of mythologies, each of which attempts to symbolize and categorize the totality of existence. By systematically exploring each category or symbol, the result for the magician is an ongoing experience of wholeness and integration. The rituals of invocation and evocation can be as simple as making a toast or can be lifetime endeavors.

Other traditions of magick are more intuitive and involve the student "seeking within" to find their path.

Above all, though, don't think of magick as a particular belief system. Think of it instead as a set of tools for managing beliefs, states, and other aspects of consciousness. Ultimately, by changing what our minds consider possible, we can change ourselves in ways that help us to adapt better to our world, to be creative, passionate, ethical, wise, or however we would like to remake ourselves. The magician is an artist as well as a scientist, working in the medium of perceptions, using the brush of the will and creating upon the canvas of the self. And in remaking ourselves, we align with the universe and change the world, too. That, of course, is a life's work. And ritual frames are a basic piece that makes much of this possible.

SETTING A SIMPLE RITUAL FRAME

1. Decide on an activity that you wish to enhance with cannabis. For instance, you might choose to get high and enjoy a walk outside, create something, make love, or contemplate and gain insight into some aspect of your life.

2. Create a simple, positively framed sentence that conveys what happens within the ritual frame. For example, "I will get high and enjoy a walk outside" is positively framed, whereas "I don't want to feel irritated" is negatively framed; it describes only what you don't want. Keep it positive. Other examples of positively framed statements include "I will get high and paint a picture of the landscape"; "We will consume cannabis together and make wonderful, transcendent love"; "I will enter a cannabis-influenced state and allow my mind to think of an idea for a new business."

3. Gather your cannabis smoking or vaporizing equipment in the place where you will begin this activity along with whatever equipment is necessary for the activity itself. Leave anything distracting or irrelevant to your activity somewhere else.

4. Say your positively framed statement out loud and then inhale your cannabis. Continue to smoke until you've reached your desired high.

5. Get immediately involved in your activity.

6. After your activity is completed, write down or record your observations.

In setting a simple ritual frame of this type, it is important to keep everything you do and say focused on your intent. That is, once you have begun, continue straight through. Don't stop to check your email, answer your phone, find out what time it is, talk about something else, etc. Develop a statement, gather your equipment, make your statement, get high, and go forth and do your activity. The frame continues to influence your consciousness until the activity is done. The retrospective act of recording your experience closes the frame and helps to later recall any important insights. For comparison purposes you might also, on separate occasions, perform your activity without the ritual frame, so you can evaluate how much it influences your experience.

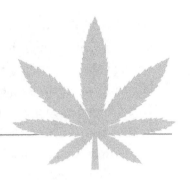

CHAPTER NINE
ENTHEOGENIC
REVOLUTION

The term "entheogen" was coined in 1979 by a group of researchers (Carl Ruck, Jonathan Ott, Richard Evans Schultes, and others) as an alternative to the word "psychedelic." Entheogen is usually defined as "god-inducing," though the researchers who first applied the term meant something more like "inspiration-inducing." While psychedelic originally had the meaning of "mind-manifesting," and referred to plants and chemicals that revealed hidden "expanded" aspects of consciousness, it shifted in meaning through popular usage to include just about anything that looked, sounded, or felt surreal or unusual. So we talk about entheogens being the plants and drugs that humans use to commune with their deities, explore their spirituality, or find inspiration. The range of things used for this purpose is somewhat wider than the set of purely psychedelic chemicals—just about anything can be used to explore spirituality or inspiration, depending on the time, place, and person.

And in fact, the time, place, and person are crucial details. When doctors Timothy Leary, Ralph Metzner, and Richard Alpert studied LSD and psilocybin at Harvard University, administering the substances to subjects under various situations, they described the important factors in determining the quality of a person's experience as *set*, *setting*, and *dosage*.

Set refers to that which the subject brings to the situation, his earlier imprinting, his learning, his temperament, his emotional, ethical and rational predilections and, perhaps most important, his immediate expectations about the drug experience.

Setting refers to the environment—social, physical, and emotional—of the session. This most important aspect of setting is the behavior, understanding, and empathy of the person or persons who first administer the drug and who remain with the taker for the period that the drug is in effect.[69]

One of Leary and company's more interesting studies along these lines (interesting, at least, for the subject at hand) is the Good Friday study. The study involved twenty divinity students, half of whom were given 30 mg of psilocybin, the effects of which were experienced during a devotional service in a private chapel on Good Friday. A placebo was distributed to the remainder of the students with neither subjects nor experimenters knowing who received which preparation. The majority of those receiving the psychedelic experienced mystical states of high quality, supporting the hypothesis that psychedelics in combination with intentionally prepared set and setting can produce quite specific results.[70] While Leary's methodology was sometimes subject to criticism, the experiment was, more recently, repeated at Johns Hopkins University with a stringent set of experimental controls—and it yielded nearly identical results.[71]

Now I hope you've noticed that the idea of "set and setting" is pretty damn similar to the concept of the ritual frame. What we are doing in either case is contriving the circumstances and programming our perceptions to produce a desired experience or outcome. Cannabis experiences are as subject to the rules of set and setting as any other entheogenic experience. In normal usage cannabis may be considered as part of the set, an element in the contrivance of

69. Leary, Timothy. "Introduction," *LSD, The Consciousness-Expanding Drug*, ed. by David Solomon, G.P. Putnam's Sons, New York, 1964, p. 13.

70. Leary, Timothy. "The Religious Experience: Its Production and Interpretation," *The Psychedelic Reader*, p. 193.

71. Griffiths et al. "Psilocybin can occasion mystical-type experiences having substantial and sustained personal meaning and spiritual significance," *Psychopharmacology*.

a ritual. That is, the herb can be used to create states of increased probability, for want of a better term, in which beliefs and certain kinds of perceptions can be willfully adopted for a purpose. Think of it at common doses as a ritual enhancer rather than center of the ritual itself.

At greater doses, especially when you eat or drink it rather than smoke, the experience can be as intense as that produced by classic hallucinogens such as the psilocybin used in the Good Friday experiments. With greatly increased intensity, the cannabis becomes more central to the ritual and the ritual elements are there to influence the outcome of the bhang trip. Either way, the outcome remains something beyond the state itself. That is, when performing cannabis-influenced ritual or ritual involving any other entheogen, the outcome is usually something other than simply "getting high" or "tripping." More typically, entheogenic rituals are intended to heal illness, commune with ancestors, yield insight, perform tasks of practical magick, and express devotion to various deities.

The act of ritualizing the use of entheogens not only intensifies the ritual itself, it places the plants and drugs themselves in a position of respect or reverence, may reduce frequency of use, and provides a level of safety for the experience. In traditional cultures that use entheogens religiously, we find that there are few social problems attributed to the sacred drugs and use remains, more frequently than not, framed as a positive, even necessary, practice. A serious ritual purpose connected with a plant will often discourage frivolous, random, or ill-considered use.

THE NATURAL GANJA RITUAL

In general, cannabis seems to have an affinity for ritual and it tends to promote natural ritual behaviors even in those who don't intentionally practice magick. It is not surprising to find that naturally evolving cannabis rituals reflect the cultural milieu in which the ritual takes place along with overall patterns that frequently parallel the consciously directed ritualizing of magick. In other words, the rituals are pretty similar whether we decided that we are doing magick ritual or "just getting high with friends."

71

Intent: Ritual often begins with a setting of intent. In a typical North American cannabis session, the idea is often enhancement of another activity, so the intent stated at the outset is often something in the order of "Let's get high and create art (or watch the sunset, play a game, have sex, sing a song, write a book, etc.)."

Participants: When it is decided that a cannabis session is about to start, invitations are given to likely participants. These participants usually must be known to the one who is doing the inviting or otherwise vouched for by another participant and must be thought of as an asset to the event. In settings where cannabis is illegal, these requirements become more stringent.

Setting: While settings are frequently improvised, they often involve finding a safe place free of distractions or interruption by nonparticipants. When cannabis is shared among several people, it tends to organize them into a circle or at least a somewhat circular arrangement. In places where cannabis is illegal, the setting needs to have a measure of secrecy about it. In choice of participants and setting, we see some behaviors that seem similar to those of "secret societies" of the past and, indeed, cannabis use is sometimes considered a sort of fraternal badge.

Tools: Special ritual tools are acquired and consecrated for use in cannabis ritual. In places where cannabis and tobacco are not generally mixed together, cannabis smoking implements are often never used to smoke anything else. Indeed, the design of cannabis pipes and rolling papers is frequently different from those used for tobacco. Vaporizers, stash containers, lighters, grinders, roach clips, and other tools are frequently consecrated for cannabis-only use.

Ritual Practices and Rules: These will vary from group to group but will often include protocols about who puffs first and second, whether the cannabis is passed clockwise or counterclockwise, how much time a participant may take for his or her turn, who is in charge of the tools, how the tools are handled, and so on.

The result is often a moderately complex multiperson ritual that is taught to newcomers and passed along over time. For example, in parts of North

America, cannabis users will typically sit in a circle, the person who supplied the cannabis will light it and take the first toke, and it will be passed to the left. This is a ritual that has been handed down to a few generations of cannabis enthusiasts and has changed little in the last forty or so years.

Other, more specific cannabis rituals have developed parallel to the group smoking circle. The best known would be the 4:20 ritual, practiced by numerous cannabis users in the US and elsewhere. The ritual began, so the legend goes, with a group called the Waldoes, students at a California university who had a meeting one day at 4:20 p.m. to go in search of cannabis plants. They never found the plants but kept the meeting time for their afternoon smoking session. The number was popularized by Steven Hager, editor of *High Times* magazine, who would arrange 4:20 a.m. smoking rituals for participants at various cannabis rallies and events.[72] The number 420 spread widely and many people treat April 20 (4/20) as a cannabis holiday.

72. Hager, Steven. *Magic, Religion, and Cannabis*. CreateSpace, 2014.

CHAPTER TEN

FREE YOURSELF FROM MENTAL SLAVERY

If set includes the beliefs and attitudes that we bring to our ritual setting, then it may do us well, first, to understand the nature of those beliefs and attitudes. What exactly rides along with us, consciously or unconsciously, when we enter our magical circle? We have beliefs that we make about ourselves, our abilities, our environment, and the nature of the world in general. Some of these are obvious; some are less obvious. Some have never quite been revealed in the light of day. Some are so basic and habitual to our world that we take them for granted.

The beliefs that we have about magick and ritual will, of course, influence the outcome of our magick. If you have a strong belief that magick is a lot of hooey and can never work, that may tend to skew your results toward failure. If you have a belief that magick is a real and powerful thing but that you have limited skills, can't learn, or always screw things up, guess what will happen with your ritual? If you are doing a ritual for prosperity but have a deep-seated belief that the economy is in ruins, that you have poor money skills, or that you don't deserve prosperity, those beliefs come with you into the circle and may manifest along with or in place of your stated intent.

It is not, however, necessary to have the opposite beliefs for your ritual to work. A useful attitude is one of possibility, an open-minded belief that, just

75

maybe, things can work out the way you intend. When you read fiction or watch a movie, hopefully you are able to suspend disbelief in a way that makes the action of the story possible. While strong belief in the outcome of a ritual may prove useful, a suspension of disbelief may produce positive results as well.

The art of always being open to possibility can be cultivated by the practice of what Robert Anton Wilson called "maybe logic." Practicing maybe logic is simple: just insert the word "maybe" after any statement of belief. "There is a god" becomes "There is a god, maybe." "The government has your best interests in mind" becomes "The government has your best interests in mind, maybe." As our perceptions are inherently limited, distorted, or flawed, there is little that we can know for sure and understanding the big *maybe* that our consciousness casts across everything we perceive can help us to negotiate the complexities of belief and possibility.

This is one place where cannabis can be useful. If we can use the cannabis state to access that kind of possibility, even just for a moment when the wild, fantastic, and otherwise unbelievable can be contemplated as possible reality, our rituals can prove more effective. Assuming that we have dispelled the limiting beliefs that we have about cannabis itself—see appendix 1 for extensive debunking of cannabis myths—we may find that our magick herb helps us to see through the conditioned beliefs and behavior patterns that define and limit our lives and may also limit our magick.

In some ascetic spiritual traditions, the aspirant—that's you—can renounce worldly things and move to the top of a mountain or to a monastery, or become a wandering mendicant. That's a fine way to isolate a meditation practice and explore it thoroughly, over time, without distraction. Sadhus renounce their former lives, give up all their possessions except a beggar's bowl and a chillum, and actively revile people and things of the consensus lifestyle. Most of us, though, want to have our spirituality and still be part of the world. We have families to care for and bills to pay. Being part of the world and still magical may be the harder path to follow, but many of us manage.

Culturally, we Westerners tend to think of cannabis as something sensual and "recreational." It certainly can be; however, in contrast, there are traditions that hold the plant as part of an ascetic path. This is something that many Western cannabis enthusiasts discover quite by accident. They may try the plant in a recreational context or to relax or for a variety of more social, sensual reasons and in the process at some point discover that the experience has disconnected them from the habits and social conventions they grew up with. This can be very disconcerting to some. In our culture, we often define ourselves by these social conventions, many of which are so fundamental to modern life that we totally take them for granted. These include such behaviors as interpersonal rapport, manners, career and work expectations, clothing styles and propriety, gender and family roles, political and ideological beliefs, and just about everything else concerning our behavior and culture. As children, we are taught social and cultural behaviors as fact: a strong handshake makes a good impression, respect your elders, it is your civic duty to vote, you call a policeman when you need help, you need to be a good provider for your family and have job security, men wear pants and women wear skirts, it is impolite to fart in company, and so on. When we experience the wider range of normally unconscious perceptions and thoughts that cannabis can bring, we suddenly realize the arbitrary quality of many of these behaviors and beliefs. We become able to contemplate other choices, alternative behaviors that might prove healthier, more fun, more useful, more fitting of our philosophical or religious beliefs, or more magical.

When consensus belief or cultural assumptions run entirely contrary to experience, then this process, called dishabituation, is furthered even more. That cannabis remains illegal and vilified while those who actually experiment with it realize its benevolence heightens the contrast of beliefs and reality. When we recognize that we have been lied to, we start to wonder about everything else. What other "facts" that we take for granted are really just propaganda? The cannabis high becomes both the subject and the means of this inquiry.

The experience of spontaneous dishabituation can be unsettling; however, once our eyes are opened to something closer to reality, we are given the opportunity to reshape our world. We choose what ideas occupy our consciousness, how we treat other people, and what we do to further our own survival.

We can make our world more interesting, exciting, arousing, beautiful, creative, compassionate, or healthy. And we can pass the attitude of open-mindedness along to others who may also be willing to make planet Earth a better place. Every act that results from dishabituation can both point the way for others who witness it and inspire freedom and happiness.

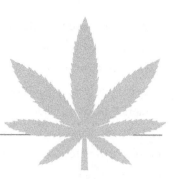

CHAPTER ELEVEN
DREADLOCKS

Thanks to modern-day Rastas, the hair nonstyle known as dreadlocks has become associated with cannabis use. In recent years, some have claimed that wearing dreadlocks is a cultural prerogative limited to Rastafari and African culture and that others would be engaged in an act of "cultural appropriation" should they let their hair grow into dreads. In fact, the association with black culture is fairly recent—indeed, until very recently African Americans who wore dreads were shunned by their own communities.[73] And the association with cannabis is far more ancient and widespread than most people realize.

Going back as far as the Scythians and the Indo-Europeans, we see depictions of dreadlock-wearing men and women in their art. The goddess of the Scythians, Tabiti, is often shown with gigantic dreadlocks. Scythian kings depicted on coins often also had dreads.

It is likely that the Scythians and Aryans brought dreadlocks to India, along with cannabis use and the worship of Indra and Shiva. (And remember, some of these people were very literally Caucasian, hailing from the actual Caucasus mountains in Central Asia.) Drawings of dread people are found in the earliest copies of the Vedas. To this day, Shiva sadhus in India grow their hair into dreads as part of their practice, rejecting the delusions and conventions of consensus

---

73. And thus, the legend goes, they were called *dread* locks.

culture. While dreadlocks were worn in Africa, it was actually Indian sailors and workers who brought the sadhu tradition of ganja and locks to Jamaica and the West Indies.

Depictions of dreadlock-wearing people can be found in the archaeological evidence of numerous ancient cultures, including the ancient Greeks, Assyrians, Babylonians, Judeans, Hittites, Chaldeans, Sufis, and many others. Photographs of nineteenth-century Native Americans show that dreads were a fairly common way of wearing hair.

The use of dreads in both sadhu and Rastafari culture represents a form of dishabituation. For the Rastas, it represents a rejection of the dominant Babylon culture. In short, most of us do not question our early training concerning our hair. We learn to comb and brush and continue to do so throughout our lives as a way of fitting into the culture in which we live. The common wisdom suggests that you have a better chance of getting a job, attracting a mate, etc., if your hair is neatly cut and combed. But that's little more than societal pressure to conform.

Along with a rejection of cultural assumptions, dreadlocks are a way of allowing your own organism to express itself in a natural way. I began this section by calling dreadlocks a nonstyle. It's how your hair grows when you leave it alone. While there are hairstyles that mimic dreads that can be time-consuming treatments at the hairdresser, real, natural dreads are created when you throw away your comb. Curly hair will lock up fastest, but everybody's hair will eventually dread if allowed to, no matter your ethnicity.

There are a variety of false beliefs associated with dreads—that they involve not washing them or the anointment of special oils or that they are difficult to maintain. In fact, dreads wash easily with shampoo like every other kind of hair, and actually will lock up faster if you wash regularly (and don't comb). Oils can help to maintain the health of hair but are not necessary for the dreads to form. And they are easy to maintain, as allowing them to maintain themselves is the point. (They do require a bit of separation when they first begin, so they don't become one single giant lock, but that's easily accomplished in a few minutes' time.)

Of course, growing dreads requires a fair amount of dishabituation and the willingness to display it to the world. You have to brave the curiosity, confusion, and occasional derision that you will get from those around you. It takes time, too. In fact, a good set of natural dreads might take a year or more to really lock up tight and the intermediary tangles and baby locks may cause even greater confusion among the denizens of Babylon.

Some Rastas and other dreadlock wearers also may hold paranormal beliefs about their hair. For some, the length and thickness of their hair recalls the biblical story of Samson, whose strength was in his locks. For others, dreadlocks are "the antenna to the universe," a connection to the wisdom and flow of their deities and nature.

Think of dreadlocks as a long-term ritual, a consecration to dishabituation, a sign to the world that you have explored and questioned your cultural conditioning. Dreads (or any specific ritual, really) are not necessary to magick, of course, but serve as an example of how we can live our lives in ways that express magical intent. What other long-term rituals might fit into your life and express your own way of being you?

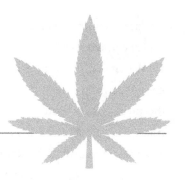

CHAPTER TWELVE

MARIJUANA
AND MEDITATION

Cannabis and meditation have been closely linked since prehistory. We've already discussed some of the history of the plant in relation to Hinduism, Taoism, and other meditation-heavy traditions. We've seen Aleister Crowley linking samadhi (a state of union that is one of the possible outcomes of meditation) with cannabis. So what exactly makes this such an important and historic connection? Let's start with some basics.

There are so many different practices labeled "meditation" that it's sometimes difficult to come up with a simple definition of the practice. For some, meditation means simply thinking about something, as in "meditate on how you ended up here, reading this book." For others, meditation might be following a guided fantasy or visualization. For the most part, though, meditation is a set of specific practices that help to quiet the mind and develop useful outcomes such as enhanced calm, relaxation, increased ability to focus, and greater awareness. In many (if not most) traditions, meditation may lead to mystical outcomes, including awareness of the unity of existence and the ability to raise and direct psychic energies.

The catch in most of these practices is that actually thinking about any of these outcomes detracts and moves attention away from meditation. Meditators are generally advised to simply meditate without desiring a particular outcome, which can be a confounding idea to goal-oriented twenty-first-century practitioners.

Wherever you might be, whatever thoughts might be in your head, acknowledge and accept what is happening and then aim your attention toward the process of meditation. And that is essentially the process: while concentrating on the object of a particular meditation—a mantra, a symbol, a chakra, a candle flame, the experience of breath or sitting—a variety of thoughts will arise. Each thought is perceived, acknowledged and then attention is returned to the meditation.

The distracting thoughts that arise can range from intrusions of minor physical discomfort ("My nose itches!") to thoughts about the day ("Will I get the project done before my boss gets upset?") to full-blown, full-sensory daydreams. In the context of meditation, these are not repressed or denied in any way. Each break in concentration, no matter what form it might take, is acknowledged, accepted for what it is, and then attention is brought back to the meditation.

Observing the ebb and flow of concentration and distraction during meditation can be enlightening in several ways. First, we are observing the interplay between the consciously focused prefrontal cortex and the brain's default network, the tendency for various parts of the brain to chatter between themselves when no conscious focus is applied. The ability to quiet the default network builds concentration ability that can be applied across many different life tasks. If you learn to concentrate at meditation, you'll also improve your concentration for reading, playing, working, or for whatever you need. Regular practice can also lessen the internal dialog and rumination characteristic of depression and anxiety, which is based in the default network.

Second, the distracting thoughts that arise may give us some indication of what kinds of things lurk below ordinary awareness. After a while, we may start to notice patterns in the kinds of thoughts. Are they mostly physical distractions? Worries about money? Fantasies about sex, food, or vacations in exotic places? Memories about childhood, friends, family, or traumatic or pleasant incidences of the past? No matter how serious or trivial the thoughts seem, they may hold clues to resolving the ongoing issues of our life. Additionally, as each thought arises in consciousness, it may be reconsolidated in memory along with some calm from the meditative state, subtly changing the way we respond to these thoughts in the future. But leave the analysis and retrospective for later and bring your attention back to the object of your meditation.

If you keep pursuing your meditation, then benefits continue. Daily practice (indeed, regular practice of almost anything) will mirror the same meditative process over time. Do you get distracted by other activities and forget your practice times occasionally? Do you sometimes get tempted to take a day off, watch TV instead, go out with friends, and so on? Just as with a break in concentration during meditation, these distractions can be acknowledged and accepted and then you turn your attention (and behavior) back to your practice.

Here are a few simple meditation techniques to explore:

SIMPLE ZEN

Sit in a position with your spine vertical and straight (a chair will do nicely). Allow your breathing to become relaxed and natural. Let it set its own rhythm and depth, however it is comfortable. Focus your attention on your breathing, on the movements of your chest and abdomen rather than on your nose and mouth. Keep your attention focused on your breathing. For some people an additional level of concentration may be helpful. You might add a simple counting rhythm spoken in your head as you breathe: "One" on the inhale, "Two" on the exhale, and repeat. Or you might visualize your breath as a swinging door, swinging in on the inhale and out on the exhale.

MINDFULNESS MEDITATION

Sit and pay attention to your posture, your breathing, and your environment. As thoughts arise in your mind, note them, give them a label, and then let them go. Label them without being judgmental. That is, note that "this is a thought about an itch"…then let it go. Or "this is an emotional thought of love [hate, anxiety, compassion, happiness, etc.]" and then let it go and return your attention to your present experience.[74]

---

74. For more information, see my book *Brain Magick*.

BASIC MANTRA MEDITATION

Select a short phrase to concentrate upon. This can be something from a spiritual tradition, an affirmation that you'd like to use, a nonsense phrase (or phrase in a language you don't understand), or simply counting. Repeat the phrase out loud (if circumstances permit) or in your head. If and when your mind wanders from the mantra, accept the distracting thought without attempting to repress it, and then, as soon as you are able, return attention fully to your mantra.

Okay, so what happens when you combine meditation with cannabis? Again, it depends somewhat on set and setting, but there are some general tendencies we can explore. Remember that cannabis has the ability to allow for both focused awareness and imagination. Meditation is usually an interplay between these, but when cannabis is involved, they can occur simultaneously. That is, you can have thoughts, see visions, hear sounds, have various feelings, and—with practice—keep focus on the object of your meditation at the same time. This allows for a unique kind of experience in which one can continue to meditate while insights and other thoughts that might otherwise be intrusive can continue to happen, too.

Meditation, in general, gives us practice in observing and participating in the normally unconscious action of our minds. Cannabis seems to intensify this process, allowing for more "second attention," the part of consciousness that can observe itself. As well, noticing the contrast between high and non-high states can reveal even more insight into our internal processes.

As with most of the practices in this book, I will suggest that it is important to be familiar with both the technique and the cannabis experience before you combine them. That is, practice your meditation regularly without cannabis so that you can ascertain what kind of experiences are, in those circumstances, typical for that technique. And be familiar with the particular kind of cannabis and route of administration that you intend to use. Then combine carefully. Start with a small amount, a puff or two if you are smoking. If it seems like more would be useful, complete your meditation session and experiment with a greater amount on another occasion.

Just about every kind of meditation or ritual will benefit from repeated practice and it may happen that the really interesting, exciting, educational, or mystical experiences will result after you have explored regularly for a while. How long? Everyone is different and times may vary, but the more you practice, the better it gets.

WATCHING THE SMOKE

This is a very basic meditation that uses smoke as the focus of attention. This can be done with incense, which will burn longer, or with the smoke from the end of a joint. Very simply, take a deep toke, then, as you breathe deeply and comfortably, hold the joint or incense in front of you at a distance of a foot or two and observe the smoke rising. Keep your head and eyes aimed forward and focus on the stream of smoke that is directly in front of you. Repeat the toke until you have reached an appropriate state, then continue observing the smoke. Allow all other thoughts to dissipate and just watch it rise. As new thoughts arise, acknowledge them, then return your attention to the observation.

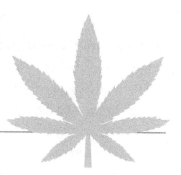

CHAPTER THIRTEEN
BREATHING

Because so many of us prefer to smoke or vaporize our cannabis, the plant and the act of breathing are connected. Newbie smokers often have a bit of a learning curve in terms of getting a full inhalation of smoke or vapor. It may take a little practice and conscious effort to get it right. Interestingly enough, there's a similar connection between breath and meditation.

Breathing is a natural link to our own unconscious processes. Usually we breathe without thinking about it; our brains and bodies keep respiration flowing smoothly along with all the other autonomic processes that keep us alive—heartbeat, digestion, endocrine function, and everything else. We can turn our attention to the other things that we do in life and, generally, we keep right on breathing. But if we want, we can change our breathing depth and rate—or just hold our breath entirely, if we choose.

Breath is also closely linked to our mental state. When we are anxious or stressed, our breathing may become shallow; when we relax, it may deepen. There are many subtleties to how we breathe, including what parts of the lungs are involved, what chest, abdominal, and back muscles we use, and so on. Each variation in the way we breathe may be related to a similarly subtle (or not so subtle) change in mood, awareness, and more.

Breath meditation, in the yoga tradition, is called pranayama, and down through the ages, yogis have explored many techniques and aspects. Here are some basic techniques:

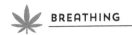

YOGIC BREATH

Your lungs have three main areas: the bottom, which is controlled by movements of the diaphragm and is visible as a rising and falling of the abdomen ("abdominal breathing"); the middle, controlled by expansion and contraction of the rib cage; and the top, controlled by the rising and falling of the shoulder blades. Each of these different kinds of breathing are associated with different states of consciousness. For purposes of the yogic breath, however, the key is simply to fill and empty *all three* of the areas of the lungs. Sit with your back straight, and fill and empty your lungs completely but smoothly, without halting or straining. This is not hyperventilation—it is proper and full breathing at a relaxed pace.

PRANAYAMA—SQUARE BREATHING

Once you are comfortable with the yogic breath, you can begin to slow it down a bit. Figure out your usual time for an exhalation or inhalation, then add one second to it. Let's say that you normally exhale a yogic breath for four seconds—you can now begin to practice pranayama by inhaling for five seconds, holding your breath in for five seconds, then exhaling for five seconds and holding your breath out for five seconds. Five in, five hold, five out, five hold—and repeat.

PRANAYAMA—CIRCULAR BREATHING

Take full, even, yogic breaths and entirely eliminate the pauses at the top and bottom of the breath so that your breathing cycle becomes a seamless and constant ebb and flow.

Notice that the yogic breath and many other forms of meditation are practiced with the spine vertical and straight. This has both practical and esoteric reasoning behind it. On the esoteric side, much of what we know about yoga here in the West comes from Tantric and kundalini-based traditions. In these traditions, the energy centers along the spine—chakras—are put into physical alignment as a precursor to their more mystical alignment. On the more practical side, good posture is generally healthy—and sitting with your spine straight allows your lungs to expand more fully. That allows for greater control of your breath—and a bigger toke, if we're talking cannabis.[75]

In the 1970s, the US was visited by a teacher from India named Baba Ganesh. Baba Ganesh was not only the leader of one of the largest Tantric orders, he was also a leader of the sadhus and an advocate for cannabis-enhanced meditation. Whenever he was asked for advice from American cannabis users or meditators, he invariably began with the same advice: keep your spine straight![76]

THE YOGIC TOKE

This is essentially the same as the yogic breath except that you use the inhalation to draw in cannabis smoke or vapor. Keep it gentle and, again, know your technique and material ahead of time to avoid coughing or other problems. Repeat until you have achieved your desired state. Note how this may change the quality of the high or other aspects of the experience.

CANNABIS PRANAYAMA

Again, this is the same as other forms of pranayama with the addition of cannabis smoke or vapor. Depending on your material, you may need to add the cannabis on only the first one to three breaths and then continue with the meditation as you would otherwise. Note how this changes the quality of the high or the experience of the meditation.

---

75. Interestingly, studies have demonstrated that cannabis users perform better than most people on pulmonary function tests. (See Pletcher MJ, Vittinghoff E, Kalhan R, et al. "Association between marijuana exposure and pulmonary function over 20 years." *JAMA*, 2012. https://www.ncbi.nlm.nih.gov/pmc/articles/PMC3840897/.)

76. Neuhaus, Eve Baumohl. *The Crazy Wisdom of Baba Ganesh: Psychedelic Sadhana, Kriya Yoga, Kundalini, and the Cosmic Energy in Man.* Inner Traditions, 2010.

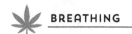

EXPANSION AND CONTRACTION BREATHING

Imagine a circle around yourself, at about the diameter of your outspread arms. Sit or stand in the center of that circle. Fill your lungs completely, with a slow, even inhalation. As you inhale, allow your attention to expand to fill the circle. As you exhale, slowly, evenly, and completely, allow your attention to contract to a single point in the center of your chest. Repeat. Do this for at least five minutes.[77]

---

77. For more information, see my book *Brain Magick*.

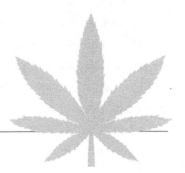

CHAPTER FOURTEEN

CANNABIS AND THE LIMBS OF YOGA

According to Patanjali, author of the ancient Yoga Sutras, there are eight "limbs" of yoga: yama, niyama, asana, pranayama, pratyahara, dharana, dhyana, and samadhi.[78] While I am generally attempting to use generic methods in this book to allow you to apply the ideas to whatever belief system(s) you work and play with, I'm going to give Patanjali and the traditional yoga terminology its due. Think of the yogic method as just that, a method, a technique that can be used by people with diverse belief system affiliations. It also provides words for concepts not found in English and will allow for discussion. And, of course, yoga and cannabis have a long-shared history.[79]

Yama and niyama, in their usual form, probably incorporate more traditional Hindu belief systems into their methods, but as Aleister Crowley

---

78. Patanjali. *The Yoga Sutras of Patanjali*. Translated and with commentary by Swami Satchidananda. Integral Yoga Publications, 2012.

79. Prior to writing this, I googled "cannabis and yoga" as part of my research and to keep up with any news. What I found, along with info about sadhus and "420 yoga classes," was a series of admonishments from the followers of "traditional" gurus with warnings such as "cannabis overheats the crown chakra," "cannabis has never been used regularly by real yogis," and "intoxicants of any kind should be avoided." The first is unproveable jargon, the second is an outright lie or ignorance of history, and the last is a valid rule within the context of some but not all systems.

pointed out, it's not necessary. Yama ("control") and niyama ("virtue") are often taken to mean a form of morality or adherence to a code of behavior, diet, etc. set forth by authorities of ancient times. Yama includes the things not to do, the "thou shalt nots" of the system, and niyama includes the positive things that we do to make our lives and the world better. We can think of yama and niyama more as living impeccably by your own code so that your life becomes more suitable for practicing yoga. That is, if you do things that run contrary to your ethical beliefs (whatever they are), it produces complications in your life and unease in your mind, all of which make concentration more difficult. If you behave in ways that are congruent and support your own beliefs about how to act, how to treat others, and how to eat right and take care of yourself, then your mind can be that much calmer when you go to practice your meditation.[80]

There are a number of yama and niyama issues associated directly with cannabis, including things like being generous and fair when sharing, buying, or selling the herb; finding safe ritual space in which to partake; using ecologically sound and sustainable agricultural practices; not walking off with someone else's lighter; creating positive ritual and meditative experiences; and so on. Even just for a regular smoking session, the yama and niyama of the practice may influence whether you enjoy or benefit from the experience. Yama and niyama are ways of influencing set.

The next two limbs are asana and pranayama, which are closer to what most people think of when we talk about about yoga. Asana concerns the physical positions that we use to meditate or move. These include the more familiar asanas of hathayoga that people learn in yoga classes, things with fun names like downward dog and pigeon pose. They also include the seated postures that are used for the more internal kinds of meditation such as lotus and half-lotus. Instructions for these are widely available on the internet or in books, so I'll skip the details except to say, "Keep your spine straight!"

The exercise-like asanas of hathayoga were, in part, derived from the Tantric tradition of raising kundalini, a latent reserve of mystical energy that arises from the base of the spine (more on that in coming chapters). Stretching and

---

80. Crowley, Aleister. *Eight Lectures on Yoga*. New Falcon, 1985.

asana are used to align the spine and clear the channels through which the kundalini energy will move. And, of course, like the gym brochure says, you'll get fit and lose weight too! The seated meditation asanas are a way of training the mind to eventually be free from the irritations and distractions of the body and allow greater concentration. (And these come with added benefits, such as fuller breathing and better digestion.)

The next limb is pranayama, breath control, which we have already discussed and practiced.

The next four limbs, pratyahara, dharana, dhyana, and samadhi, are equal parts method and result. Arising from the preceding practices, the state of pratyahara is one in which the mind is turned completely inward and the meditator loses awareness of the external world. I'm not aware of any neuroimaging studies of the pratyahara experience, but this does seem like an interplay between the intent of executive function and some aspects of the default network. The internal landscape, as it were, is usually a default network creation and pratyahara places it, to a greater extent, under the conscious direction of the meditator.

This is a good thing, because the next limb is dharana, which means "concentration." This is where we officially meet the meditation method that we've been discussing all along. This is the process of concentration interrupted by the wandering mind and then returning to concentration. The part of it that is intentional method is the act of concentration and the result includes the interrupting thoughts. Both are considered part of dharana and it is the interplay between them that teaches us about the habits of our minds, eventually quiets the default network, and, with continued practice, leads to the next limb.

That next limb is dhyana, which is meditation itself, complete and unbroken concentration on the object of meditation. The meditator forgets entirely that he is sitting on a rug in an ashram, having chosen to do these crazy things, and there is nothing but the object of concentration.

As the identification with the object of meditation deepens, ego dissolves and we experience the eighth limb of yoga, samadhi, the state of mystical union in which subject and object merge and all is perceived as one.

These latter limbs are difficult to describe by their nature, which has in part led to the general perception of pratyahara, dharana, dhyana, and samadhi as rare states that are granted only to great mystics, sages, and gurus. In fact, these are natural and fairly common experiences. We experience the inward-directed experience of pratyahara in daydreams, while reading poetry or fiction, and sometimes when we lose ourselves in work. We experience the process of concentration/wandering mind/concentration whenever we attempt to focus our attention, whether that might be studying, playing music, memorizing something, or whatever might require our extended attention. And many people do experience flashes of unity on the level of samadhi while in flow states, during ecstatic group events like concerts or raves, sometimes during sex, and sometimes from the use of entheogens. These are all natural tendencies of the human mind. The trick with meditation is learning how to explore, extend, and enter these states intentionally.

And, to get to the point of this discussion, all of these states can be experienced spontaneously while using cannabis. It's not a given that they will be, of course; the rules of set and setting apply. But many people have their first tastes of these states while high. Albert Hofmann, among others, theorized that yoga (and other religious and spiritual techniques) may have originated as an attempt to recreate the experiences produced by the nectar of the gods, amrita, which upon reaching the earth became the magick herb of Indra and Shiva, cannabis.[81]

Stay tuned! More cannabis yoga techniques coming up in the next chapter.

---

81. Schultes et al., 2001.

CHAPTER FIFTEEN

ENERGY MEDICINE

U p to this point, science has been a useful ally. While we'll continue to take hints from the consensus body of knowledge and from the methods of science, we're about to take a few steps into the unknown. There are phenomena described by humans in almost every culture, time, and place on planet Earth that science has yet to fully explore. Yes, we are about to enter a realm of possibility, of experiences that might be mystical woo-woo or that might prove to be future science. Consider these ideas as the basis for experiments—and form your own theories.

A concept that appears in the belief systems associated with many different forms of meditation, martial arts, magick, and healing practices is the idea of a life force energy, called "ch'i" in Chinese systems, "ki" in Japanese systems, "prana" in Indian systems, "ashe" in African diaspora traditions, and various other names in other practices.

There are those who take this energy to mean a kind of cosmic energy that pervades everything. Fritjof Capra in *The Tao of Physics* relates ch'i to the quantum field, describing both as "a tenuous and non-perceptible form of matter."[82] The Eastern sources, however, are almost bewildering in the diversity of definitions

---

82. Capra, Fritjof. *The Tao of Physics: An Exploration of the Parallels Between Modern Physics and Eastern Mysticism.* Shambhala, 2010.

applied to ch'i. Ch'i is the life force energy, but it is also inner energy, intrinsic energy, and even focus of attention.

In the eight-circuit model of consciousness developed by Tim Leary, Robert Anton Wilson, and others, the awareness of energy in and around the human body is attributed to the neurosomatic circuit. The neurosomatic circuit is the fifth of the eight circuits and the first of the four emergent circuits, the abilities and experiences that humans are evolving into.[83] Each of the circuits may be activated by a particular drug, and the specific drug that Leary and Wilson associated with the neurosomatic circuit was, yes indeed, cannabis!

> The phenomena of "faith healing," "regeneration," "rejuvenation," bliss, ecstasy, rapture, etc. have been occurring for many thousands of years, in all known cultures. In the pre-scientific language of yesterday's psychology we would refer to such events as "psychosomatic." In our deliberately modernistic and almost sci-fi jargon, we prefer to call them *neurosomatic.*
>
> The neurosomatic circuit of the brain is much more recent than the antique circuits previously discussed. It does not manifest in all human beings, and appears late in life, usually, to those who do activate and imprint it.
>
> *Temporary* neurosomatic consciousness can be acquired by (a) the yoga practice of *pranayama* breathing and (b) for those who can handle it, by ingestion of Cannabis drugs, such as hashish and marijuana, which trigger neurotransmitters that activate this circuit...
>
> ...Pranayama creates neurosomatic Turn On: *sensory* enrichment, *sensual* bliss, *perceptual* delight, and a general laid-back Hedonic "high." Similar effects are produced by *voluntary* isolation in a Lilly tank, by zero-gravity (the astronaut's "mystical" experiences are all of this neu-

---

83. The first four circuits are *bio-survival, mammalian-territorial, semantic,* and *socio-sexual* circuts, which all humans have imprinted to one degree or another. The "upper" four circuits, *neurosomatic, neurogenetic, meta-programming,* and *quantum non-local* are appearing in some but not all humans. Please note that the circuits describe behavioral imprints and are not to be confused with the chakras, Sephirah, or aspects of any other system.

rosomatic variety) and, for the judicious or lucky, Cannabis drugs, as said above.[84]

So, as widespread as these experiences may be, we don't fully understand the experience of energy itself. Are there real but previously undetected energy fields around the human body? Is it the quantum field, as suggested by Capra? Is it a metaphor for subtle and mostly unconscious perceptions? Or is it some combination of these—or something else entirely?

Wilson notes that neurosomatic experiences are not limited by linear, one-thing-at-a-time thought processes. Thought, perception, and understanding seem to happen in gestalts, complex systems and aggregations of thought. In a more usual context, we use some of these gestalts to understand other humans: our unconscious minds process the nonverbal cues of someone, perhaps a smile, posture, breathing patterns, hand gestures, etc.; we put them all together; and we intuit whether the person is happy or sad, angry, distracted, focused, high, ecstatic, etc.

The experience of these gestalts is generally accepted on a conversational level, if not on a mainstream scientific level. We usually accept the idea that "willpower" or "will to live" can make the difference between success and failure, survival and death in many situations. We often accept that some people can influence others simply "by force of will," "power of belief," or "energy level" (i.e., "His level of energy is so high that he inspires everyone around him!").

So one simple way to understand energy is as a gestalt of consciousness itself. It is the focus of attention and all that includes—the pictures that people create and look at both internally and externally, the sounds and voices they listen to internally and externally, the feelings they are aware of both internally and externally, and the tastes and smells they can either experience or imagine. If you pay attention, you quickly learn that everyone sorts images (and sounds and feelings) in space around them and inside them. While they (and you) may not characterize these images as such, they pretty closely match the various phenomena ascribed to ch'i. That is, if a person's attention is fixed in one area of their body, they will manifest symptoms, abilities, weaknesses, and

---

84. Wilson, Robert Anton. *Prometheus Rising*. New Falcon, Hilaritas Press, 2016.

strengths directly related to how they are visualizing that body part. If a person's attention is fixed outside the body, and spread out over a number of different visualizations, they will, as you might expect, act scattered, spaced out, or uncentered. If they are strongly focused on a particular activity or subject, they will tend to have strong abilities (or weakness) in that activity, depending on how and what their visualization includes.

The Eastern systems of meditation and martial arts have extremely refined methods for focusing ch'i—that is, for directing attention in useful ways. While much of this has not been verified (or even tested, for that matter) by Western science, it has been practiced and studied in the East for thousands of years. In yoga, for instance, the chakras mark areas of the body in which energy (prana) can be concentrated by meditation with specific effects derived by that practice. If you focus and maintain your attention in a particular chakra, you can develop abilities, experiences, and states of consciousness that are consistent with other people who similarly concentrate their attention. In Chinese systems, the meridians also mark flows and localizations of ch'i in the body. If an acupuncturist's needle draws consciousness to a particular point on a meridian, consistent effects will be produced.

BECOMING AWARE OF ENERGY

First note where you habitually place your attention. Is it concentrated in one area or areas? Is it all over the place? Does it form a particular shape? Is it more in some parts of your body than others? Once you've mapped where you usually keep your ch'i, you can experiment by surrounding yourself with imaginary geometric figures—cubes, spheres, pyramids—and let your awareness, the aura of your perception and attention, take those shapes. Do you experience different subjective feelings? Do you have different kinds of thoughts while using different shapes? Are some shapes easier for you to practice with than others? Do factors like symmetry and balance play a part in how the shapes feel?

Now get high and repeat the experiment. How does your experience change? Do you feel comfortable with the same shapes or different ones?

BASIC CHAKRA ACTIVATION

There are seven chakras running in a line from the base of the spine to just above the top of the head. Some people imagine them as lotuses placed along the spine or as glowing vortices of light in front of the body, with tails that enter the body and connect to the spinal cord. Sitting with spine straight, imagine each chakra in turn while you take three yogic breaths and intone (either out loud or in your head) the appropriate mantra.

The chakra at the very base of the spine is red and the mantra is "lam."

A few inches above that, the chakra is orange and the sound is "vam."

At the solar plexus, it is yellow and "ram."

The heart chakra, in the center of the chest, is green and the sound is "yam."

The throat chakra is blue and the mantra is "ham."

Above that, the third eye chakra is indigo and the sound is "aum."

The crown chakra, just above the top of the head, is violet and is observed in silence.

CHAKRAS AND SMOKE ACTIVATION

Take a large inhalation of smoke or vapor before chanting each chakra, imagining the smoke flowing into the chakra. Then chant the appropriate sound at least three times before moving on to the next chakra. Notice how this may change the experience of the chakra meditation—and how the chakra meditation can change the experience of getting high.

PARTNER CHAKRAS

Perform the same exercise with a partner, concentrating on and chanting the sound for each chakra together. Experiment with positions: sit next to each other, both facing the same way; sit back-to-back with chakras aligned; sit face-to-face with chakras aligned; or, if consensual, sit in a Tantric yabyum position.

After completing the meditation, take some time to sit together and notice how you feel, what thoughts come to mind, and so forth. How does working with a partner change the experience?

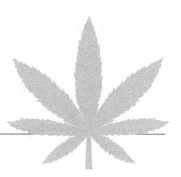

CHAPTER SIXTEEN
KUNDALINI

In some schools of yoga, kundalini represents a special case of the life force energy. This is the postulated reservoir of energy that sits at the base of the spine, waiting to rise up through the chakras, through the top of the head, to create an energetic union with the universe at large. Again, the theorizing here borders into the realm of woo-woo, but kundalini itself appears to be a real phenomenon, reported by numerous yoga practitioners as well as psychonauts who spontaneously experience nearly identical sensations while using entheogens. Other extreme experiences may trigger kundalini experiences, including accidents, trauma, childbirth, or orgasm.

Kundalini is most often experienced as an intense vibration or bright light that moves up the spine. It may be accompanied by various sounds and physical sensations of heat, cold, pain, pleasure, and bliss. The rush of energy may also bring unexpected insights, realizations, and movements. At its peak, especially during initial encounters, it can result in a lapse of consciousness.

In Tantric Buddhism, cannabis is referred to as "food of kundalini" and is consumed as a bhang beverage prior to kundalini-raising rituals, which are often sexual in nature.[85] In Hindu lore, kundalini is symbolized as the union between the goddess Shakti and her lover Shiva. Remember him? Lord of yoga? The god who gave ganja to humankind? When Shiva was purifying the amrita,

---

85. Ratsch, 2001.

it was a snake that assisted him, the symbol of kundalini. Yoga and cannabis seem to be magically suited to combine and stimulate kundalini experiences.[86]

There are several theories about the nature and origin of kundalini. Some writers have speculated that it is a physical wave or spasm in the cerebrospinal fluid that surrounds the spinal cord. Others speculate that it is caused by release of endogenous psychedelic chemicals in the body. Dimethyltryptamine (DMT), which may be produced in the pineal gland along with other tryptamine chemicals such as melatonin, is considered a leading suspect.[87] A recent study that compared the experiences of DMT users with reports of near-death experiences (NDE) tends to confirm the close similarity of the psychedelic experience with NDE.

Another suspect would be potassium ions and other chemicals that block glutamate receptor sites. This was proposed by researcher Dr. Karl Jansen, who was studying the glutamate receptor–blocking drug ketamine. While studying a proposed link between ketamine experiences and non-drug-related near-death experiences, Jansen noticed that some ketamine trip descriptions were remarkably like traditional descriptions of kundalini.[88] Large enough doses of DMT would likely also cause glutamate blockade effects.

And, of course, so would large doses of cannabis. Recent studies have demonstrated that the CB1 cannabinoid receptor plays a central role in moderating glutamate receptors. Too much glutamate released during trauma or stress can be toxic to the nervous system, so a natural process of blocking the receptors may be a protective adaptation, a way to save the brain from burning out during extreme situations. Again, we see the moderating effect of the endocannabinoid system, charged with maintaining balance throughout the

---

86. This will be a controversial idea for followers of "traditional" gurus who eschew drug use of any kind. On one hand, exploring these powerful and challenging experiences without drugs is encouraged prior to combining them and abstinence may be excellent advice for some people, at certain stages of life. On the other hand, the "drugs are bad, m'kay" attitude has been adopted by some of these schools as a way of fitting in and seeming more respectable to Western audiences, even though the gurus are surely aware of the long-shared history of yoga and cannabis.

87. Strassman, Rick. *DMT: The Spirit Molecule: A Doctor's Revolutionary Research into the Biology of Near Death and Mystical Experiences*. Park Street Press, 2001.

88. Jansen, Karl. *Ketamine: Dreams and Realities*. MAPS, 2001.

various systems of the body. These various theories are not mutually exclusive; the cerebrospinal fluid contains a variety of endocannabinoid chemicals and may respond to their release with a wave-like movement.[89] The systems of yoga familiar to practitioners in the US are generally derived from traditional forms that were part of kundalini practice. The most common type of yoga, the hathayoga exercises that are taught in gyms and yoga studios everywhere, were originally for the purpose of clearing the energy channels and preparing the body for the arousal of kundalini. A lot of attention was (and is) paid to the flexibility and correct posture of the spine. (Sit up straight!) The best-known systems of yoga meditation, chakra meditation, and Raja Yoga in general, are for the purpose of bringing the energy up through the cleared channels. (Note that the two supporting channels, ida and pingala, are often depicted as twin serpents climbing the channel that runs up the spinal column, a symbol sometimes found carved into hemp stalks, suggesting some relationship between cannabis, kundalini, and, perhaps, the staff-and-serpent symbol of Aesculapius, which has become our modern symbol for medicine.)[90]

Just as someone may have a bad trip from a psychedelic, it is also possible to have unpleasant kundalini and neurosomatic experiences. Most famously, the Indian writer Gopi Krishna recounts how his kundalini meditation sent him into a painful and traumatic period of his life (though when he eventually passed through that period, the kundalini became a source of bliss that he sought to share with the world).[91] Robert Anton Wilson maintained that many (but not all) of those who activate the neurosomatic circuit will undergo a visit to Chapel Perilous, a dark night of the soul—essentially an extended and intense bad trip. For some, this "crossing the abyss" is a form of radical dishabituation, a reality check of epic proportions. The unpleasantness may be a habitual holding-on to the beliefs and behaviors accumulated up to that point in life. It can be very painful and difficult to release beliefs about who we are,

89. Kantae et al. "Quantitative profiling of endocannabinoids and related N-acylethanolamines in human CSF using nano LC-MS/MS" *Journal of Lipid Research*, Volume 58, 2017; Rodríguez-Muñoz et al. "Endocannabinoid control of glutamate NMDA receptors: the therapeutic potential and consequences of dysfunction." *Oncotarget*, 2016.

90. Clarke and Merlin, 2013.

91. Krishna, Gopi. *Kundalini: The Evolutionary Energy in Man.* Shambhala, 1997.

our role in the world, and how we relate to others. To realize, all at once, how many of these beliefs were randomly acquired and ill-suited to our nature can seem like the world is crumbling around us.[92]

I might suggest here that if kundalini is a part of your intent or practice, you then keep the concepts of set and setting firmly in mind, even if you are "just meditating." These "bad trips" via kundalini, much like psychedelic trips, may prove to be powerful life-changing learning experiences or a kind of shamanic initiation.[93] As such, it may be worthwhile to enlist the help of an experienced teacher, coach, or guide to help navigate through the shamanic underworld.

The techniques for working with kundalini have already been described, primarily pranayama, hathayoga, and chakra meditation. Those alone can induce kundalini experiences—and the addition of cannabis increases the likelihood of it happening.

Now the question remains: Just what is kundalini good for? I'm still working on an answer to that, even after thirty plus years of kundalini experiences. The guru Sri Chinmoy suggested that kundalini made one capable of amazing feats of strength, and well into his eighties, Chinmoy would give demonstrations in which he would lift thousand pound weights. Some practitioners claim that kundalini gives hands-on healing ability, personal health and longevity, and new, creative ideas. Personally, the only things I've noticed following kundalini experiences are insights into my yoga practice itself (that is, what asanas and how to practice them, among other things) and a general tendency to be happier. I would attribute both, I think, to the novelty and intensity of the experiences, factors that help to stimulate neuroplasticity and neurogenesis in the brain.[94]

---

92. Wilson, 2016.

93. Ibid.

94. For more information, see my book *Brain Magick*.

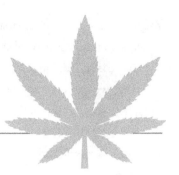

CHAPTER SEVENTEEN

HYPNOSIS

As we've noted, the cannabis experience is one of the rare states in which both executive function and the default network can be accessed simultaneously. The set of experiences closest to cannabis might be found via the techniques of hypnosis. As with meditation and magick, this isn't a new idea, and the association of hypnosis and cannabis may go back a long way, perhaps to the Egyptian temples of sleep, which probably employed an early form of hypnosis.

James Braid, considered one of the seminal figures in modern hypnosis and the person who coined the term "hypnotism" in the nineteenth century, made a study of hashish use and noted the similarity with hypnotic, magical, and psychological phenomena.[95] Much later and more infamously, US intelligence agencies in the precursors to the better-known MK-ULTRA program found that a combination of a high dose of cannabis and hypnosis was the closest thing to a truth serum that they could produce.[96]

A popular conception of hypnosis isolates it in the psychotherapist's office, in some kind of occult setting, or in the performance of a stage hypnotist. While early theories of hypnosis were based on mystical mesmeric fluid or animal

95. Braid, James. *The Discovery of Hypnosis: The Complete Writings of James Braid, the Father of Hypnotherapy*. National Council for Hypnotherapy, June 2009.

96. Lee, Martin A., and Bruce Shlain. *Acid Dreams: The Complete Social History of LSD*. Grove Press, 1994.

magnetism, a modern understanding of the field treats hypnotic phenomena as a process that utilizes natural shifts in our language and perception.

There is no hard and fast definition for a hypnotic experience or trance. The best that we can do is to say that a trance state is an altered state of consciousness, one that represents a shift from "ordinary" waking consciousness. Some emphasis has been given to the ideas that a trance state represents a more internalized experience, a narrowing of focus, dissociation, increased suggestibility, or automatism. While any of these can come into play in a hypnotic experience, none of them are either necessary or universal. Perhaps one of the most useful definitions of hypnosis is "a goal-directed striving which takes place in an altered psychological state."[97] Speaking of hypnosis in the context of a therapeutic setting, Milton Erickson wrote, "Trance permits the operator to evoke in a controlled manner the same mental mechanisms that are operative spontaneously in everyday life."[98]

Notice that both of these quotes, written before there was a well-developed field of neuroscience, can be understood as references to the relationship between the default and executive function modes of the brain. Ronald Shor's "goal-directed striving" would be an aspect of executive function, and the altered state would involve the internal experience of the default network. And given Milton Erickson's hypnotic style, the "mental mechanisms" of which he wrote would be the ones that allow switching between the two major brain modes.

As we are able to observe some of the action of the default network, it may be easier to understand that our minds have the ability to shift from one state of consciousness to another very easily. We have all experienced trance-like states while daydreaming, bored in a lecture or class, driving along a long highway, getting a massage, sitting in a hot tub, shifting our attention in order to read an article or book, watching television, or going inside our own minds to think about something.

There are many, many methods of hypnosis and self-hypnosis. For a long time, some researchers used a kind of statistical approach to studying hypno-

---

97. Shor, Ronald E. *Amer. J. Psychology*, Vol. 13, 1959, 582–602.

98. Paper credited "circa 1960s" first published in *Hypnotic Investigation of Psychodynamic Processes, The Collected Papers of Milton H. Erickson, vol. III.* Irvington Publishers, 1984.

sis. That is, they would take one method of inducing trance and apply it to a large group of test subjects. The results, invariably, would "prove" that only a percentage of the population were "good hypnotic subjects." In fact, all that was really demonstrated was that that particular method of hypnosis was effective with a percentage of the population. In the 1960s and '70s, Milton Erickson began publishing papers on his inquiries into hypnotherapy. Erickson proposed a new model of hypnosis that suggested that trance states could be accessed quickly and easily in everyone by using flexible trance inductions that developed a biofeedback loop between the therapist and patient. That is, Erickson would incorporate observable aspects of the client's experience and feed them back to the client in a variety of ways. He would, for instance, match the rhythm of his voice to the client's breathing or heart rate, while describing with his language other verifiable aspects of the client's experience such as the way they were sitting, any movements they made, what they were looking at, etc. The observable aspects could then be tied to less verifiable "leading" suggestions; for instance, Erickson might gently slow the rhythm of his speech while saying, "As you breathe…like this…you can become…more relaxed." The tendency is for the patient to follow into the suggested states. This was a dramatic departure from the predominant hypnotic methods of the time that were more directive and less permissive.

Erickson's techniques can be applied to self-hypnosis as well as the therapist/client situation. The following, developed by Milton Erickson's wife, Betty, according to legend,[99] is a simple method of self-hypnosis that can be learned and practiced quickly:

THE BETTY ERICKSON TECHNIQUE

Sitting comfortably with eyes open or closed, list to yourself three things you can see, then three things you can hear, then three things you can feel (for example, "I see the color of the wall, I see the person opposite me, I see the color of her hair, I hear the sounds outside the room, I hear people moving about, I hear my own breathing, I feel the cushion underneath me, I feel the air on

---

99. It is taught with this title in numerous hypnosis courses and books around the world, although an original source written by Mrs. Erickson cannot be found.

my skin, I feel my hands on my lap…"). Then narrow it down to a list of two things in each sensory mode and one thing in each mode. Tell yourself, "As I count from ten down to one, I can go into a deep, comfortable trance." Then count breaths backward from ten to one and enjoy the trance that you are drifting into. This works most powerfully when the verbal listing within your head is timed in rhythm with your breathing.

Practice this a few times (on different days) without cannabis. Notice what the trance experience is like. Notice whatever similarities and differences to the cannabis experience you can. Then (on another day) practice after you get high. Notice any differences in the experience. Are parts of it more or less intense, relaxing, or unusual?

While cannabis in the popular imagination is thought of as something that interferes with memory, in reality it can be very useful for recall of long-term or even long-lost memories. The similar properties of hypnotic trance are also often used for this purpose—and the combination of cannabis and hypnosis can be a very powerful way to reexperience aspects of past times and remembered places. Again, it is recommended that the following exercise be practiced at least a time or two without cannabis, to familiarize yourself with the technique and the experience, before combining.

HYPNOTIC MEMORIES

1. Identify a particularly relaxing or enjoyable experience.
2. Recall what you saw there, what colors were present, whether it was bright or dark, what objects were in your field of vision, whether there was motion or stillness in what you saw.
3. Recall what you heard there, what kind of tone the sounds had, whether it was loud or quiet, rhythmic or not.
4. Recall what you felt at the time, the temperature of the air, what position your body was in, what your skin felt like, what kind of emotional or internal feelings you may have had.
5. Recall what you tasted or smelled at the time, whether it was sweet or sour or bitter, strong or mild.

6. Run through each sense and increase the intensity in your mind—make the colors brighter, the sounds clearer or louder, the feelings stronger.

7. Enjoy your experience and explore it in whatever way is comfortable. This kind of suggestion can be used in a therapeutic or medical context to help a patient relax in the face of what might otherwise be an anxiety-producing situation. By accessing a past state when the patient was more relaxed or had a reduced heart rate or lower blood pressure, it may also be possible to help the patient reexperience the physical parameters of that memory as well as the mental. The suggestions can be incorporated into a conversational context or can be marked out to isolate a "relaxation experience." As with anything else, practice is required, though these techniques are simple enough that they can yield effective results very quickly.

A particularly useful aspect of this kind of recall is that you can recall and reexperience altered states as well as mundane memories. This happens quite naturally sometimes. When I presented this technique at the Starwood Festival, many years ago, I was approached afterward by Stephen Gaskin, who related to me that he often didn't actually have to smoke his herb, but would get very high just looking at it, smelling it, and rolling a joint.

The key to this kind of recall is what we call anchoring. That is, we use sensory cues that are either naturally occurring or deliberately created that serve to recall the state. The sensory cues need not represent all the senses, but starting with one kind (usually kinesthetic cues—feelings) can serve to help recall all associated sensory experiences. That is, by recalling the way cannabis makes you feel, you can often reexperience much of the complete high.

WEED OF CHOICE PATTERN
(RECALLING A HIGH)

Recall a time when you were pleasantly high. Remember where you were, whatever that place was like. Take some time to recall what you did to get high, starting at the beginning; for instance, opening a bag, crushing a bud, smelling the herb, the feel of it in your fingers, the way it felt to roll a joint (or whatever you did), the way the joint felt in your hand, and so on, up to and including smoking,

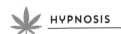

vaping, etc. At that point, recall how it felt as the effects first became noticeable. Then, track the kinesthetics of the experience as follows:

1. Notice where in your body the feeling of the state begins.
2. Notice where it moves to as the experience develops toward its peak.
   Pay attention to whether the feeling is moving or static, cycling or pulsing.
3. Give the feeling a color. "If this feeling had a color, what would it be?"
4. Apply the color everywhere you have the feeling, creating a three-dimensional colored shape.
5. Experiment by making the colored shape brighter, darker, richer, faded, larger, or smaller to determine which of these increases the feeling associated with the state.
6. Notice any other changes in feeling as well as in what you might see, hear, taste, or smell.
   When you have accessed the desired state, enjoy it and make use of it in whatever way you choose. Afterward take some time to think about what aspects of the experience were more difficult to access, what aspects were easier to access, and how the experience was similar to or different from the original experience.

Another useful aspect of this kind of hypnotic process is that you can take present experiences and enhance or tweak them in various ways.

ENHANCING A HIGH

This begins much like the previous exercise, except instead of using a memory, take some time to get high in the present. Smoke, vape, eat, or whatever you do and when you have reached the desired state, map the experience by following the internal physical sensations:

1. Notice where in your body the feeling of the state begins.
2. Notice where it moves to as the experience develops toward its peak.
3. Pay attention to whether the feeling is moving or static, cycling or pulsing.
4. Give the feeling a color. "If this feeling had a color, what would it be?"

5. Apply the color everywhere you have the feeling, creating a three-dimensional colored shape.

6. Experiment by making the colored shape brighter, darker, richer, faded, larger, or smaller to determine which of these increases the feeling associated with the state.

7. Notice if the colored shape is cycling or pulsing (usually as you breathe). If it is, you can accentuate the cycle or pulse, expanding it and moving it through your whole body.

8. Add some special effects to your color(s). These can include sparkles, auras, shimmers, diffraction, or whatever helps to further intensify the experience.

9. Enjoy and make use of the resulting state for ritual, meditation, activity enhancement, relaxation, or fun.

THE IMAGINARY JOINT

This is a group experiment that can offer insights into cannabis rituals when it is practiced in a few different ways. Practice (1) with a group that has never smoked or vaped together, (2) with a group that regularly gets high together, and (3) if possible, with a mix of experienced cannabis users and participants who have never used cannabis.

Very simply, have everyone act as if a real joint is being prepared and smoked. Items like rolling papers, trays, grinders, and lighters can be employed as they usually are—but with only imaginary cannabis. Imagine and act out every detail you can think of—opening the bag, smelling the herb, the feeling of crushing a bud between fingers, using a grinder, rolling the joint, lighting it, passing it around, toking, holding it, exhaling, etc. (Pass around an entirely imaginary joint; put the real rolling papers, etc., away after the imaginary joint has been created.)

After you have imagined that the joint has burned all the way down, take a moment to notice how you feel, what the other participants are doing or saying, and anything else of note. If you were able to practice this with different groups of people, as described above, how were the sessions different?

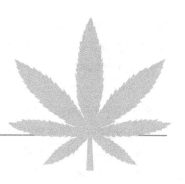

CHAPTER EIGHTEEN

CONTACT HIGHS AND SHARED EXPERIENCE

Milton Erickson was once asked if he went into trance as well when he induced trance in a client. He responded that he went into trance *first* and then took the client with him. As with many of Erickson's techniques, he was capitalizing on a natural tendency of human consciousness. We are often influenced, subtly or overtly, by the people around us. This is something natural that we've all experienced. Think about that wet blanket friend whose sullen demeanor brings down the whole room or that upbeat person who brightens a room when they enter.

An extreme version of this phenomenon is called shaktipat by the yogis. This is when the mere presence of a guru or enlightened person confers enlightenment on someone else. It can also be used to describe spontaneous kundalini experiences that are stimulated by the presence of someone with aroused kundalini.

And this kind of experience-sharing happens among cannabis users. Friends who have not consumed any herb will act high, silly, humorous, or philosophical when hanging around with their pothead buddies. Of course, it can happen with other substances, too, especially the psychedelics; a few people on LSD or MDMA can change the consciousness of an entire crowd at a concert or rave.

Nor is it strictly limited to drug experiences—as Dr. Erickson suggested, almost any state can be conveyed nonverbally, either spontaneously or by intent.

Becoming aware of this process can be useful in a variety of ways. If you have the ability to shift the consciousness of others, you can help them get out of stuck or unpleasant states. You can get a group of ritual participants into the same headspace. And you can also protect yourself from inadvertently taking on the negative states and feelings of others.

When we do this kind of thing intentionally, the process is called pacing and leading and relies on the brain's mirror neuron system. Mirror neurons are motor neurons that respond not only when we decide to make a movement but when we observe (or hear, feel, or even think about) someone else moving. When the mirror neuron system registers sentient activity that we are familiar with—movements that we have made ourselves or are presently making—it responds more strongly. For instance, if a couch potato watches a martial arts film, s/he can experience some of the action and may be moved to imitate some of the techniques, however ineptly—but if an experienced martial artist watches the same film, her mirror neurons respond more strongly and any internal or external imitation will be much more detailed. Likewise if an untrained rock 'n' roll fan hears a great guitar riff, he might be moved to play some air guitar, but if an experienced guitarist hears the same riff, her air guitar will include more accurate finger and hand movements and more nuances of hearing.

When we see, hear, or feel others who are behaving like us, we experience greater empathy and rapport. Rapport, on the most obvious level, is a feeling of comfort or trust that we have while communicating with other humans. An easy way to think of rapport is as a kind of resonance. We fall in step with each other, harmonize, see eye-to-eye. Neurolinguistic programming (NLP) techniques to develop and maintain rapport include a process of matching or mirroring behavioral cues. You have undoubtedly noticed how this can happen spontaneously: one person yawns, so does her friend; in a classroom of silent test-takers, one person coughs and it spreads around the room; when friends hang out together, one person laughing can infect the others with giggles. The matching and mirroring, called pacing, tends to develop both comfort and trust.[100]

There are a lot of subtleties to pacing and leading, in fact the more subtle, the more effective. Matching obvious movements can be fairly effective (especially if you're doing something like dancing or making love); however, matching unconscious movements can be even more effective. That is, if you can identify some movements or behaviors that are outside of someone's awareness and match or mirror them, your rapport may develop even more rapidly and deeply. Some unconscious behaviors are easy to observe like breathing, eye movements, and facial expressions.

Once you feel that you have some measure of rapport, you can then change your behavior to lead into a new state or movement. If the shifts are smaller, natural, relaxed, and within the person's normal range of behavior, they tend to compel more than abrupt and unusual behaviors.

While this process can seem awkward when we first attempt to practice it intentionally, it is the same process that happens naturally and outside of awareness in cases of contact high and in many other situations. At least a little bit of dishabituation may be necessary to move these very habitual and unconscious behaviors into consciousness. A good way to start is by observing others. Notice how good friends tend to fall into the same postures and movements when they are hanging out together. Notice how it sometimes takes one willful person to change their behavior to motivate a group of people who are in deep rapport (for instance, the first friend to stand up and say, "Hey, we'd better get going if we want to make it to the movie on time!"). Also notice how people who are in the same state of consciousness, like those getting high together, tend to find rapport more easily and naturally.

INTENTIONAL CONTACT HIGH

Find a friend who may need a little relaxation, pain relief, euphoria, or a case of the munchies. Get high and then go sit or stand with your friend. Without drawing attention to what you are doing (that is, do what you normally do

---

100. Carey, Benedict. "You Remind Me of Me," *The New York Times*. February 12, 2008. http://www.nytimes.com/2008/02/12/health/12mimic.html?_r=1.

in a similar situation—chat, eat, watch TV, or whatever), match your friend's breathing and some aspects of posture and facial expression. Take at least a few minutes and notice when it starts to feel comfortable, then relax and start to explore your high. Go with the feeling of being high and allow your muscles to soften, your breathing to change, and your mood to lift (or whatever really characterizes the high for you). Enhance the experience by using the Enhancing a High exercise from the previous chapter, if necessary. Notice whether your friend is following you into the state (that is, observe any changes in breathing, posture, facial expression, behavior). If you need to, return to pacing to deepen rapport, then lead some more, until you've transmitted a nice contact high.

As mentioned, there are numerous uses for this technique. If friends or ritual partners all engage in this kind of rapport-building with each other, it can be a powerful and consensual experience. Some people will think of more nefarious ways to attempt to influence others covertly. While that is possible using similar techniques, it's not as easy as it might seem. Remember that rapport works both ways. When you develop rapport with someone, it's not just other people feeling comfortable and trusting around you—if you've got a functioning set of mirror neurons, you will likely also feel that way about them! And I'll also mention that when dealing with rapport, there is no substitute for authenticity. That is, it all works best when you are genuinely interested and well-intentioned toward the people you hope to influence.

Unusual things can happen when people are in rapport together, including the appearance of some very unordinary abilities and phenomena. In the 1950s through 1970s, research into parapsychology was a little bit more mainstream than it is today. Researchers at quite a few universities actively pursued links between hypnosis and parapsychological phenomena. While it can be argued that none of the studies could point to a conclusive and easily replicable result of ESP, in many of the studies, the subjects who were asked to make guesses scored higher after a hypnotic induction. Not for every subject or every single trial of the more successful subjects, but over dozens of studies by different researchers, the scores following trance techniques averaged out significantly higher. A meta-analysis of the numerous individual studies of hypnosis and

ESP concluded that "It seems that the difference in ESP performances in the induction and control conditions is a reliable effect—it occurs more often than would be expected by chance and it does not appear to be due to faulty ESP testing or experimental design."[101]

A more recent experiment by Canadian neuroscientist Michael Persinger may provide a clue to the phenomena. Persinger is best known as the developer of the "God Helmet," a device that uses mild electromagnetic stimulation to activate the temporal lobes. Most who try the helmet report an altered state and many report significant or transcendent experiences of various kinds. The use of transcranial magnetic stimulation is well-established—you can go to a neurologist's office for TMS treatment for a variety of neurological problems, for instance. What is remarkable is one of the experiments to which Persinger applied his brain machine. He had two subjects in different rooms, each with their own helmets. They could not see or hear each other. Their only connection was the computer that controlled both helmets, so that both would be in the same state simultaneously. After both had spent some time with the helmets, Persinger came into one of the rooms with a flashlight, which he aimed at the subject's eyes. Predictably, the subject's eyes reacted, the pupil contracting. What is strange is that in the other room where there was no flashlight, the other subject's pupils also contracted at the same time.[102]

This is more like the kind of result one sees in quantum physics, where particles that were once connected continue to influence each other instantly at a distance. Persinger has theorized that his experiment demonstrated quantum entanglement on a human scale. Fascinated with the experiment, I asked two of my online classes to see if they could develop a low-tech version of the experiment as it might relate to "spooky action at a distance," as Einstein called it. The result was an experiment that resembled the old hypnosis and ESP studies as much as it did Persinger's helmet-entanglement project. Here are the instructions for the initial trials of one of the experimental groups:

101. Rao, K. Ramakrishna. *Basic Research in Parapsychology, 2nd ed*. MacFarland, 2001.

102. Hu, H. and M. Wu. "Transatlantic Excess Brain Correlations Are Experimentally Produced by Persinger's Group." *Journal of Consciousness Exploration and Research*, Volume 6, Issue 9, September 2015.

We'll conduct this experiment a number of times, with changes in one variable, that variable will be the state that we are in when we test. To start with, however, the first round of testing will be with NO particular state. Or rather, whatever state you are in when you come to the test, without any special preparation.

I am going to lift up one of my limbs, right arm, left arm, right leg, or left leg. I'm going to concentrate on that limb for a full minute. I will repeat this at least three times throughout the day.

Now … without any preparation, just as you are reading this now, make a guess as to which limb. There are four possible answers—right or left arm, right or left leg. Make a guess and then post it here.

When each one of us has guessed (or remote viewed, or intuited, if you prefer), then someone else will concentrate on one of their limbs and we will repeat with the same parameters until each of us has had a turn as "sender." So … timing on this will be dependent on time zones and when people can get online to test, but let's see if we can move through this part of the experiment quickly.

The other class used a nearly identical system but employed playing cards for the guesses. In the first trial of the arm/leg experiment there were no attempts to control state. In subsequent trials we had both senders and receivers employ the same methods for state control. The first method was to yawn ten times. And right away, our correct guess scores began to improve. The next state control method was the yoga meditation technique of square breathing and our scores shot up even higher! The playing card class also found that their guess scores increased dramatically when state control techniques were shared.

This experiment is low-tech enough that if you have access to a computer and a group of friends, colleagues, or students, you can replicate it for yourself using meditation, hypnosis techniques—or cannabis! While this is a very preliminary and homebrewed kind of experiment, it demonstrates at least the possibility that sharing states may also share other, less overt aspects of consciousness. And if that's the case, think about what happens with a group of people getting high together. There are multiple elements of ritual that go into creating communal states—and the addition of a bit of cannabis passed around may deepen connections and depth of interaction. And the phenomenon of the contact high suggests that the joint doesn't even have to make it all the way around the circle; a few high participants can help to develop a shared state in a larger group.

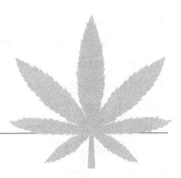

CHAPTER NINETEEN
LAUGHTER

Any discussion of shared states has to mention the one behavior that reveals or develops rapport faster and deeper than most. No, we're not talking about sex. We're talking about laughter.

Most of us, hopefully, have noticed that when we laugh with someone, we feel closer and more comfortable with them. (If you haven't noticed this in your life, grab your best friend and get your butt out to a comedy show or a funny movie. Do it right now! What are you waiting for? These are important life experiences!) This may be because the laughter reveals a preexisting rapport. Or it may be that the simultaneous behavior is a variety of pacing. And laughter not only denotes a state, it can generate one as well—and the shared state may help connect consciousness on a deeper, more mysterious level.

One thing we know about cannabis is that it can bring the laughter. In fact, two of the names for cannabis in the Vedas, the ancient antecedents to Hinduism, are *vijahia*, source of happiness, and *ananda*, laughter-provoker.[103]

In general, laughter is good for you. Very good for you, in fact. There are a few neurological conditions that can cause "sham laughter," an unpleasant and uncontrollable symptom that sounds just like normal laughter, but that's a bit different than the genuine kind that we experience when we hear a joke or see something funny. That kind, the funny kind of laughter, has a variety of health

---

103. Bennett, 2010; When the first endocannabinoid was discovered, it was named Anandamide.

benefits. Laughter increases healthy blood flow, it oxygenates the brain, it lowers levels of the "stress hormones" cortisol and epinephrine, it stimulates the release of pain-relieving endorphins, and it strengthens the immune system.

Norman Cousins, who coined the phrase "laughter is the best medicine," claimed to have cured a serious connective tissue disease with laughter. Given a one in five hundred chance of recovery from the extremely painful condition, Cousins developed his own treatment routine that involved watching Marx Brothers[104] comedies and the old *Candid Camera* television show. He found that ten minutes of deep belly laughter could give him two hours of pain-free sleep—and he eventually recovered.[105]

There are a number of theories about why we laugh. A popular theory is that it evolved from the sense of relief that we feel when we escape from danger. As such, it is a relief of tension. Laughter also acts as an important social cue. Again, it is an indication of rapport, and if we accept the "escape from danger" theory, it may signal a shared sense of relief and perhaps a bit of interpersonal bonding for the mutual defense against future danger. This theory suggests that a joke presents a moment of confusion or ambiguity, and as we figure it out, we have a sense of relief that it doesn't represent danger.

A related theory was offered by a professor I had in a college class titled "English Composition: Humor." He claimed that all humor involved a reaction to pain, a defense mechanism perhaps, and he challenged us to find examples of humor that are not at someone's expense. When I posed this idea to author and general funny person Paul Krassner, he said, "No ... I think it's all a matter of scale. A tickle is actually a gentle form of pain, and you can take that all the way up to humor in the concentration camp, as Benigni does in the movie *Life Is Beautiful*. But back to my original no. I always resist when college professors generalize. Humor can relieve tension, but tension isn't necessarily painful.

---

104. Chico Marx claimed that his brother Groucho got his name from the "grouch bag" that he habitually carried. What was a grouch bag? Something in which you kept a little bit of marijuana.

105. Cousins, Norman. *Anatomy of an Illness As Perceived by the Patient*, 20th Anniversary Edition. W. W. Norton, 2005.

Consider your various bodily functions that function on tension. Now *that's* funny."

Laughter may also provide opportunities for dishabituation. When I discussed this with comedian George Carlin, he told me, "When a person is laughing, they are defenseless. It is a completely zen moment. You are never more yourself than when you have been surprised into laughing. That is a moment when your defenses are down, in a manner of speaking. Most of the time, when you talk to people about…let's call them "issues," okay? People have their defenses up. They are going to defend their point of view, the thing they're used to, the ideas that they hold dear, and you have to take a long, logical route to get through to them, generally. This is all generalization. But when you are doing comedy or humor, people are open, and when the moment of laughter comes, their guard is down, so new data can be introduced more easily at that moment."

Some spiritual and religious traditions make use of this principle to free minds and bring enlightenment. This includes the numerous jokes of Zen and the often mind-bending humor of Sufi stories. The legendary Sufi storyteller, jokester, fool, and sage Mullah Nasrudin is considered (if we accept that he was an actual person, not merely a literary character) as the creator of the modern joke and the author of many "old jokes" that are still around today. He might be the one to blame for all the amusing musing about roads and the motivation of chickens.

In some traditions, humor is the central element, for instance Discordianism or the Church of the SubGenius. Discordianism proposes a doctrine that includes the "Curse of Greyface":

In the year 1166 BC, a malcontented hunchbrain by the name of Greyface, got it into his head that the universe was as humorless as he, and he began to teach that play was sinful because it contradicted the ways of Serious Order. "Look at all the order around you," he said. And from that, he deluded honest men to believe that reality was a straightjacket affair and not the happy romance as men had known it.

It is not presently understood why men were so gullible at that particular time, for absolutely no one thought to observe all the disorder around them and conclude just the opposite. But anyway, Greyface and his followers took the game of playing at life more seriously than they took life itself and were known even to destroy other living beings whose ways of life differed from their own.

The unfortunate result of this is that mankind has since been suffering from a psychological and spiritual imbalance. Imbalance causes frustration, and frustration causes fear. And fear makes for a bad trip. Man has been on a bad trip for a long time now.

It is called THE CURSE OF GREYFACE.[106]

Of course, the way to banish the Curse of Greyface is simply to laugh at the humorless bastard.

A central tenet of the Church of the SubGenius is, in the words of their legendary founder, J. R. "Bob" Dobbs: "Fuck 'em if they can't take a joke."[107]

Banishing by laughter is also a practice of chaos magicians, another good example of using natural, spontaneous behaviors in a more conscious, intentional way. We often say we're able to "laugh it off" or, in retrospect, look back and laugh. Used intentionally, a good laugh will change your state and will reframe whatever is being laughed at in a less threatening way. The intention of a banishing is to clear your mind and your working space and a laugh can easily do the first and can serve as a symbolic way of doing the latter. In chaos magic, one technique is to create a magical sigil that expresses a particular outcome and then to find a way to consciously forget about it, and laughter (along with other methods such as burning or tearing up the sigil) can assist by creating a sudden shift in consciousness.

---

106. Malaclypse the Younger and Omar Khayyam Ravenhurst. *Principia Discordia*. CreateSpace, 2011.

107. Stang, Ivan and The SubGenius Foundation. *The Book of the SubGenius: The Sacred Teachings of J.R. "Bob" Dobbs*. Touchstone, 1987; Another saying of "Bob" is "If you think it's a joke, you don't get it!"

Chaos magicians also do funny (but real) rituals that invoke Harpo Marx.[108] And, in the spirit of Harpo, one person will often be appointed to inject humor into whatever group rituals are being practiced, to keep egos from running amok and prevent stultifying seriousness.

Some people take laughing yoga very seriously. Yes, laughing yoga is a real thing! While jokes and humor are allowed, laughing yoga usually starts with "voluntary laughter." In other words, laughing yogis "fake it 'til they make it" by acting out a good laugh, until the group laughter becomes contagious and genuine. Along with exercises to develop group rapport and playfulness, the actual laughing part becomes a group pace and lead that takes everyone to the funny place. Studies have demonstrated the kind of health benefits that you would expect from spontaneous, genuine laughter, including improved mood and cardiovascular health. While we have begun to see "420 yoga" sessions in places where cannabis has been legalized, these are, as far as I know, hathayoga classes and so far there aren't any 420 laughing yoga sessions, except for the natural kind that somehow seem to happen around 4:20 p.m. anyway.

LAUGHING EXERCISE #1

In the spirit of Norman Cousins (with a dash of Tommy Chong), get high and watch a Marx Brothers movie. *Duck Soup* and *A Night at the Opera* are highly recommended. Afterward, take a few moments to think about how you feel.

VOLUNTARY LAUGHTER

Perform a few minutes of voluntary laughter, preferably with a friend or two. First do it with no cannabis; then, on a separate occasion, get high and do the same thing. After each session, take a few moments to check in with your body and mind and notice how you feel and what your mind may be doing. Notice what happens when you just laugh; notice what (if anything) changes when you get high first.

---

108. Hine, Phil. "Mass of Chaos 'H.'" https://www.chaosmatrix.org/library/chaos/rites/cmassh.html.

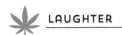
LAUGHTER WITH INTENT

Think about some quality you can use more of in your life, for instance, passion, wisdom, patience, intelligence, courage, relaxation, empowerment, creativity, or whatever you choose. Make it a positive quality (rather than a negative for which you might say "I don't want *x*" or "I want to *x* less," make it something positive for which you can state "I want *x*"). Think about what it would be like to have more of that quality. Remember any times that you had as much of that quality as you ever did. Or think about someone you know who has a lot of that quality and imagine what that would feel like. Imagine having that quality in abundance; feel it in your body. Then, as you allow the feeling to build, let it come out as a laugh that expresses the quality. Remember how to make that laugh. Then let the feeling fade; go do something else for a little while to clear your mental palette. Lastly, just make the laugh, as you did previously (though without the buildup of memories, etc.) and notice how much of the quality and state return.

Later, experiment with this laugh and this entire process when you are high. Notice if it is easier to access and build up the quality/states and how easily the feelings return.

LAUGHTER PACING

Get high with a good friend. In the course of your normal interactions, get your friend to laugh. When they do laugh, join in. If you can, match the tonality, rhythm, volume, and general sound of their laugh. Notice which of these factors tends to stimulate more laughter in your friend. Continue to pace their laughing and prolong it as much as you can.

LAUGHTER BANISHING

Make an imagined visual image of some factors in your life that you could use less of, that unpleasantly occupy your mind, or that you, generally, need to change your attitude about. You can use images of actual events/situations/people in your life or create a symbol for those situations, similar to the Discordian Greyface. Holding the image(s) in front of you, laugh at them, deep and long. A "laugh with intent" can be used, or just give it a good belly laugh. Notice what happens to the images when you do this. Afterward, take a moment to think about these factors and notice how your thoughts and feelings about them have changed.

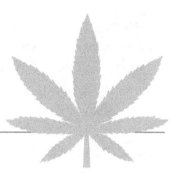

CHAPTER TWENTY

HEALING

Before we get into this chapter, I'd like to mention that I believe that cannabis and "psychic healing" can be wonderfully effective, especially when used as a complement to the care and treatment from a medical doctor, but this by no means replaces a doctor! If you're sick, see your doctor first!

In the New Testament it is told that Jesus performed a variety of miraculous healings, even raising Lazarus from the dead. He also turned his disciples loose among the people to perform healings. The biblical accounts suggest that some of the healing feats in these stories were a property of the cannabis-based holy anointing oil that Jesus may have distributed to his flock.[109] And the New Testament is far from the oldest account of cannabis-related healing, nor is it the first in the historical record that documents even more miraculous methods. We find similar stories of hands-on healing throughout world history.

The earliest pharmacopoeia all include cannabis as an important medicine, a tradition that continued down to (almost) modern times when cannabis tinctures and medicines were available over the counter until marijuana prohibition began in the US in 1937. We've already addressed the importance of the endocannabinoid system and how cannabinoid chemicals help to maintain the dynamic balance of the various systems of the body. By encouraging homeostasis, the

---

109. Bennett, 2010.

balance of all the systems and processes in your body, cannabis can act as a powerful medicine and can reset many aspects of the organism. There are also some important allopathic effects of cannabis, including improved metabolism and insulin resistance (important in treating diabetes),[110] bronchodilation (important in treating asthma and other respiratory problems),[111] lower ocular pressure (which helps to treat glaucoma),[112] antitumor effects (important as an adjunct in cancer therapy),[113] and much more.[114] Cannabis can also activate the healing processes associated with laughter.

There are at least a couple other related healing mechanisms that can act in concert with the pharmacological and humor-inducing aspects of the herb. These are at the less-studied, more magical end of the healing spectrum: energy healing and belief change.

We've already discussed the reality-selection properties of the cannabis experience. At the level of the individual neuron, cannabinoids signal whether a new neural pathway is strengthened or deleted. Ultimately, the collection of all such strengthened neural pathways defines how we perceive and respond to the world around us. At the level of observable thought and behavior, cannabis gives us greater access to the super-position of choices that eventually result in

---

110. Di Marzo, Vincenzo et al. "Cannabinoids and Endocannabinoids in Metabolic Disorders With Focus On Diabetes." *Handbook of Experimental Pharmacology*, 2011, 75–104. https://www.unboundmedicine.com/medline/citation/21484568/abstract/Cannabinoids_and_Endocannabinoids_in_Metabolic_Disorders_with_Focus_on_Diabetes_.

111. Pini, A. et al. "The role of cannabinoids in inflammatory modulation of allergic respiratory disorders, inflammatory pain and ischemic stroke." *Curr Drug Targets*, June 13, 2012, 984–93. https://www.ncbi.nlm.nih.gov/pubmed/22420307.

112. Pertwee, Roger. "Targeting the endocannabinoid system with cannabinoid receptor agonists: pharmacological strategies and therapeutic possibilities," *Philosophical Transactions of the Royal Society B: Biological Sciences.* http://doi.org/10.1098/rstb.2011.0381.

113. Velasco Diez, Gulillermo et al., "Anti-tumoral effects of cannabinoid combinations," patent application, GW Pharma LTD [GB]; Otsuka Pharma Co LTD [JP]. https://worldwide.espacenet.com/publicationDetails/description?CC=TW&NR=201002315A&KC=A&FT=D&ND=3&date=20100116&DB=EPODOC&locale=en_EP.

114. Granny Storm Crow's List of Cannabis News and Studies. https://grannystormcrowslist.wordpress.com/the-list/.

the new neural pathways. In short, there's a state of possibility, suspension of disbelief, and an openness to new ideas and beliefs.

Dr. Andrew Weil characterized cannabis as an "active placebo,"[115] a substance that has definite pharmacological effects that also support the actions of set and setting, belief, and expectation. If your set includes the belief that something will heal, the placebo effect suggests that it will heal. The effects of cannabis let you know that *something* is happening, and if your beliefs are aligned, you can accept that what is happening is the healing that was intended. One way of thinking about this is that cannabis makes the placebo effect more noticeable and reliable.

So along with the actual pharmacological healing properties of the herb, cannabis can heal by helping to create and manage the sense of possibility and the belief in that healing—which sounds like it could be a description of the much-derided practice called faith healing.

There are numerous methods that are used to create hands-on healing. Some are honest and likely effective. Some are scams—sort of. The most basic sort of faith healing scam uses what hypnotists call convincer strategies. That is, a situation or experience is created in which the subject becomes convinced that healing is taking place. This is not unlike the action of an active placebo—*something* is happening and because of the frame in which we encounter it, we can accept that what is happening is the intended healing. A strong belief that develops in this way can trigger a placebo response and cause real healing.

One often-seen method used by televangelists is more like a stage hypnosis routine than a system of healing. The preacher touches or gestures at a person and suddenly they feel weak or off-balance and they fall to the floor. To the audience (and maybe to the subject, too), it looks like the power of the preacher has knocked them over. In actuality it is a simple hypnotic technique that creates a unique feeling in the body and, if directed that way, weakness in the legs

115. Weil, Andrew. *The Natural Mind: A Revolutionary Approach to the Drug Problem*. Mariner Books, 2004.

that allows the person to be knocked over easily.[116] The hypnotic technique it-self has little to do with healing, except that it can convince the subject of the power of the preacher (or the preacher's favorite deity) and develop a belief that healing is taking place … a belief that can, itself, heal.

Other examples of trickery leading to belief and healing can be found in the classic shaman's sleight of hand trick, seemingly removing an evil object from the subject. A more involved form of this might be the psychic surgeons who perform simulated surgery and "remove" all kinds of unusual objects and substances from the subjects. Again, it's sleight of hand with an extra helping of theatrics, but some subjects do report healing.

More honest healing methods can be found in the fields of energy medi-cine, kinesiology, Touch for Health, Reiki, EFT, and others. These variously in-volve running attention along energy meridians, touching or tapping, massage, visualization of symbols in chakras, and similar techniques. While some not yet fully understood energy may be responsible for some of the effects, part of it may have to do with attention being directed to various parts of the body in particular ways.

Studies have demonstrated that giving attention to something that is hap-pening to your body increases blood flow to those regions, while ignoring or being distracted from whatever is happening reduces blood flow.[117] Simply put, if you concentrate on part of your body, more blood will flow to that part. More blood makes an area of the body warmer, more oxygenated, better sup-plied with neurotransmitters, better able to flush toxins, and so on. Combine this healing effect with a strong belief that healing will happen and seemingly miraculous things can occur.

Of course we are, once again, talking about neurosomatic energy, all of which suggests that cannabis may be a key to real and deep healing using these techniques.

---

116. See my DVD set *How to be a Megalomaniac* (Hawk Ridge Productions, 2000) for demonstra-tions and instructions on how to do this yourself. It's a very impressive trick at parties and useful if you want to start your own cult.

117. Meyer et al. "Attention modulates somatosensory cerebral blood flow response to vibrot-actile stimulation as measured by positron emission tomography." *Annals of Neurology*, Volume 29, Issue 4, 1991.

BASIC ENERGY HEALING

Healing Yourself

Clear your space and your mind in whatever way is appropriate. Get high with your preferred method. Take a few minutes and simply sit or lie and, with eyes open or closed, become aware of your body—not only the problem area but the whole system. Take a few yogic breaths. As you continue to scan your body, notice how you represent it to yourself in your mind's eye. Do different areas feel differently? Does your mind assign different colors to different areas of the body? Or vibrations and sounds? Notice the difference in how you perceive relatively healthy parts of your system compared with the problem area(s). Is there a particular feeling or color or sound that is associated with health? Focus on the problem area and allow that healthy feeling, color, or sound to flow into that area. Notice as the healthy perceptions fill that area. The method of meditation applies—if you break concentration, acknowledge the break and return to concentration. When you begin to tire or it becomes more difficult to keep the good energy flowing, then stop. Practice pranayama for a few minutes, then rest and notice any differences in how you feel.

Healing Others

Clear your mind and space as best you can. If appropriate and acceptable, both healer and the person to be healed can get high. If it's not appropriate for both, then just the healer can partake. Increase rapport by pacing breath or other unconscious aspects of behavior. The healer then takes a few moments to practice pranayama or a trance induction technique. When a deeper altered state has been achieved, the healer sits quietly and, with eyes open or closed, scans the person to be healed. Simply allow your awareness to move from the person's head down to their toes and back. Notice any impressions, colors, feelings, sounds, vibrations, etc., that you experience as you do this. Notice how it feels/looks/sounds when you scan healthy parts of the body and how it is different in the problem area. Then, breathing deeply and comfortably, concentrate on the subject's problem area and imagine it filling with a flow of good energy that matches the energy in healthy areas of their body. Again, the method of meditation applies, and when you tire or find the concentration more difficult, then stop, breathe deeply for a few minutes, and rest. At this point, you can ask the person to be healed how they feel and if they notice any differences.

The Healing Yourself and Healing Others exercises can be practiced as often as necessary. It's a good idea to only work on others when they agree to the healing and you are feeling healthy yourself. Check in with your own feelings and with the feelings of the others being healed and make sure that you or they are continuing to improve. And, again, consult a medical doctor for any chronic or recurring problems.

Of course, there are many more complicated methods and systems of energy healing. Most do not discuss the use of cannabis as a way to enhance the techniques,[118] so I will repeat my general suggestion for exploration: learn the techniques without cannabis first, then combine carefully.

118. Although some systems, such as ayurveda, include cannabis as an important and useful medicine.

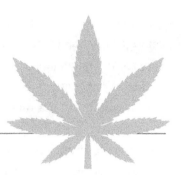

CHAPTER TWENTY-ONE

ENTITIES

Some of the earliest references to cannabis in ancient literature claim that use of the herb confers a unique power: the ability to communicate with spirits. For the most part, modern readers take that with a large grain of salt. Spirits? What? Aside from the few competing father-figure gods familiar to most people in our culture, we usually discount the idea of spirits entirely.

But magicians of yore—and many in modern times as well—summoned or spoke to gods, goddesses, angels, demons, servitors, spirits, elementals, djinni, loas, orishas, and incorporeal critters of every type. However, it's not necessary to believe in ghosts, gnomes, or unicorns—or a father god in the sky, for that matter—if you want to practice magick. Rather than unquestioned belief, sometimes all that is necessary is suspension of disbelief. If you think of the idea of spirits and entities as a thought experiment and play along as if it were true, strangely enough, you'll get results.

We actually deal with entities all the time. Sometimes we know it's all imagination, as when we read a novel and learn from a fictional character. In our minds, Sherlock Holmes remains a great detective and an inspiration to real, nonfictional detectives everywhere (and to mystery writers) even though he once only existed in the mind of Arthur Conan Doyle. Santa Claus comes and delights children (and provides seasonal jobs for both elves and adult humans) every year, and whether or not we believe that reindeer can fly, Mr. Claus still influences the behavior (and dress!) of countless actual humans.

Some of us treat our machines and devices as entities. Have you ever encouraged your car to start? Pleaded with your computer to go faster? Seriously, who are you talking to?

Identifying entities is a function of the brain's mirror neuron system, which, before it starts making you yawn or play air guitar, has to decide if something is worth mirroring. That is, does the behavior come from a sentient entity or from a brick wall? The mirror neurons use a few different kinds of cues to determine entity-hood. On the visual level, facial features and hand movements help the brain decide something is human. Coherent language, semantics, and the transmission of understandable ideas—or sounds that seem like language and ideas that seem like maybe you could understand them—are auditory clues to sentience.

One very important quality that helps the brain decide if something is an entity or not is the idea of holism. That is, does the entity comprise a complete system? In magical terms, does it have all the elements? Arthur Koestler called such whole systems "holons," and when we find them in the world around us, we tend to grant them some measure of entity-hood.

The brain and its mirror neurons can be fooled and in ways that we often enjoy. For instance, we look at cartoons, and because they have humanoid features and can communicate, we can empathize with the characters for at least the duration of the comic strip or show. Historically, car sales have done well with vehicles that have some humanoid features, such as headlights-and-grill faces in the front, and very poorly with less facey cars such as Buckminster Fuller's Dymaxion or the Ford Edsel. And humans have long attributed sentience to forces of nature and nonhuman phenomena of many types.

Some atheists make the argument that sentience is a product of the brain and that forces of nature and incorporeal entities and spirits do not have brains and therefore cannot be sentient. First, we really don't know the origins of consciousness. There are good arguments for consciousness being a ubiquitous property of the universe and brains being akin to radio receivers tuning in consciousness for the individual. Second, even if consciousness is limited to biological brains, these entities do in fact have them. They have our brains! Just as Sherlock Holmes shared Arthur Conan Doyle's brain—and the brains of everyone else who ever wrote a Holmes tale, directed or acted in a Holmes movie, read a Holmes story, or watched one of those movies—gods, goddesses, and that whole crew can easily share brains with multiple humans.

In one sense, we share brains all the time with our own various personalities. Most of us are not the same person most of the time. We have an area in the right parietal lobe of the brain that attempts to convince us that we are always, you know, *us*. But in fact, different states of consciousness are pretty much like different personalities. Are you the same person taking a test in school as you are at a rave on a Saturday night? Are you the same person early in the morning before you have coffee and later in the day when you are at work? Based on your behavior, someone who didn't know you well might not think so.

An extreme example of this is the mental illness known as multiple personality disorder, in which some people have a collection of very different personalities that have no memory of being the other personalities. Recently, brain scan studies have demonstrated that these are, in fact, discrete personalities and they sometimes do arise simultaneously in the brain without being aware of each other. This has been argued as support for the Gaia hypothesis, the idea that Earth as a whole is a sentient entity and we are all, in a sense, its multiple personalities. If, however, we can be subentities in the greater Gaia entity, then it is fair to speculate that there are other subentities, some larger than human minds, some existing as aggregations of human minds, and perhaps some entirely nonhuman intelligences.[119]

Interestingly for our purposes, entities and entheogenic plants have been associated since prehistory. On one hand, the plants are said to be tools to enable contact with spirits, gods, power animals, etc.; on the other hand, the plants themselves are considered intelligences. We call them allies, teachers, and "flesh of the gods." We give them names: *Salvia divinorum* is called *Ska Maria Pastora* by the Mazatecs, which translates to "the herb of Maria the Shepherdess"—or "Sally" by modern devotees; MDMA is "Molly"; psilocybian mushrooms were *teōnanācatl* to the ancient Mesoamericans, which translates

---

119. Kastrup et al. "Could Multiple Personality Disorder Explain Life, the Universe, and Everything?" *Scientific American*, June 2018.

to "flesh of the gods"; the spirit of opium was Morpheus, god of sleep; and, of course, among the many names and entities associated with cannabis we mostly call her Mary Jane, "Marijuana."

Magicians and cannabis enthusiasts have described a fair number of cannabis entities including some of the ones we visited earlier, like Shiva, Ma Gu, Khidr, Dionysus (a Thracian cannabis entity, before the Greeks turned him to wine), and many more. Is it all one cannabis spirit? Or does each plant or each encounter yield a different entity?

CONTACTING THE PLANT SPIRIT

While we may come in contact with a cannabis spirit every time we encounter the plant, by approaching her in a ritual context, we may have the opportunity to learn and deepen our relationship with the entity. The following ritual is one such approach.

1. Banish your ritual space with expansion and contraction breathing or a banishing ritual of your choice.

2. Consume cannabis in whatever way is safest and most effective for you.

3. Pay attention to the way the cannabis makes you feel inside. There may also be visual, auditory, olfactory, or gustatory perceptions at the same time; for now pay attention to the feeling. Pay very careful attention to how it makes you feel, the structure of the feeling. Where does the feeling start? What kind of feeling is it? Where does it go as it develops? Does it continue to move? Is it static? Follow it through to its peak. Then ask yourself "If this feeling had a color, what would it be?" Imagine the color (or colors) in your body in exactly the areas where the feeling is experienced.

4. Then imagine that you are taking the colored shape out of your body and flip it around to face you. Place it on the floor outside your circle and breathe deeply, feeding it breath and energy on each exhalation.

5. Keep breathing and feeding it energy until it transforms. The entity may change size, shape, position, movement, brightness, color, or any other factor. Once it has transformed, imagine you are communicating with it. Ask it what it wants to be called. Ask it what it can teach you that it has

never before revealed. Ask it how you can feel really good more often or how you can apply its wisdom in your life. Ask about specific situations in your life that you hope to learn about. Ask how you might use cannabis in your explorations of conscious, magick, meditation, or spiritual work. Find out whatever you can from it. Thank it for everything.

6. Closing—Absorb the entity and anything else you may have created in your aura during this operation.

7. Repeat the banishing.

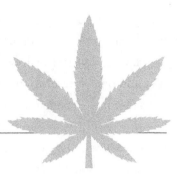

CHAPTER TWENTY-TWO
ANCESTORS

Did your ancestors get high? Maybe you know of a few older family members who enjoyed cannabis, or maybe no one else in your immediate family gets high. Either way, given the ubiquity of cannabis in the ancient world, it's likely that somewhere along the line some of your ancestors were cannabis enthusiasts or ritual users, or they ate, wore, or lit their lamps with cannabis. My own ancestors, way back when, were Scythians, which explains a few things. The Scythians conquered and settled in large parts of Europe, Asia, and the Middle East, so there's probably a lot of that going around.

Recent advances in genetics and epigenetics suggest that we not only inherit physical traits such as eye color and size, we also may pass along habits and experiences. While some of these studies only addressed fear as an epigenetic trait that can be passed down to successive generations as phobias,[120] it is certainly possible that other complex behaviors are transmitted as well.

And there's also the more obvious way in which behaviors are carried through the generations: traditions. We learn rituals, ethics, and lifestyles from our immediate family and peers—who learned it from theirs, who learned it from... etc. While cannabis use specifically may have ceased to be passed along due to lack of availability (ancestors who migrated to where there was none, for instance) and shifts in customs, some of those traditions, as we've seen,

---

120. Callaway, Ewen. "Fearful Memories Haunt Mouse Descendents." *Nature*, December, 2013.

may yet slyly point to cannabis as something our forebears revered. We may intuit a blank spot, a hole in the traditions, perhaps, which we feel moved to fill.

Magical and spiritual traditions throughout the world pay special attention and offer reverence to the ancestors. This includes Judeo-Christian traditions that may include remembrance rituals (Yahrzeit in Judaism, for instance), holidays paying tribute to particular dead people (the presidents' birthdays or Catholic saint's days, for example), holidays to connect with ancestors (Roman Catholic All Soul's Day, or the Mexican Day of the Dead) and adaptations of Pagan ancestor rituals (Halloween).

We are the culmination of everything our ancestors were and did. In a sense, they remain a part of us—and we are part of the greater collection of minds in which they also participated. That's a strong connection and accounts for an awful lot of information that might be passed down to us. And there may be even stronger links. Remember the "contact high" experiment in which two people in the same state were in rapport even when not physically together? Does the same kind of quantum link (as Persinger hypothesized) work through time as well as space? If we get high now, does that create a link to all our ancestors who were cannabis enthusiasts?

More than one ancient culture believed so. The use of cannabis as a means to communicate with ancestors dates back to Paleolithic times.[121] In ancient Korean traditions, we find shamanic use of cannabis to contact ancestors and spirits and also the use of hemp in funeral rituals. The corpse is dressed in hemp cloth and hemp is used in various other ritual trappings. This suggests the creation of a link between the hempen deceased and the hemp-inspired shamans.[122] We find this idea more explicitly practiced in various parts of Africa, including Rwanda, where cannabis incense is burned to contact ancestors who also enjoyed the herb.[123]

---

121. Clarke and Merlin, 2013.

122. Ibid.

123. Ratsch, 2001.

Cannabis was used in funeral traditions including the Korean and Scythian rites already discussed, and many others. Along with a possible link to the ancestors, the herb may have a more immediate application to funerals. The endocannabinoid system helps us to control some emotional processes and may be very important in moving beyond trauma. The key may be in the unique property of cannabis to help us forget. As well, getting high keeps our attention in the present and influences memory consolidation toward calmer, more useful states. So popping your head into a Scythian hotbox tent and catching a good lungful of cannabis vapor might be a good way to integrate and transcend grief.

In states where cannabis is legal, we are already seeing cannabis-friendly weddings in which the traditional consumption of alcohol is replaced with fine herb. In coming years we may see a similar trend in wakes and funerals when cannabis is returned to its ancient ritual use.

In some African diaspora traditions, the earth, the soil that we walk upon, is considered to *be* the ancestors. It's a good observation in low-tech societies where bodies are not embalmed. Instead, the bodies decompose and reunite with the soil. In turn, plants grow from the soil and we eat, drink, and smoke those plants. Another aspect of ancestors that is explicit in African traditions, we find that some of the ancestors become legends and the legends elevate them to the status of loas, orishas, gods, and goddesses. For instance, Chango was a great king and warrior; his legend became entwined with the legends of other great kings and warriors, and over time, he came to be thought of as a loa or orisha, the voodoo and Santeria equivalents of deity.[124]

It's likely that other gods and goddesses that we've already discussed here became divine through a similar process. The story of Jesus may have been based on a living rabbi of the time (and conflated with the legend of Mithra, among others). Notably for our purposes, Indra and Shiva may once have been

---

124. Scranton, Laird. "Shango: Yoruba Diety," *Encyclopedia Britannica*. https://www.britannica.com/topic/Shango; Duncan, Cynthia. "Chango, Lord of Fire and Lightning," *About Santeria*. http://www.aboutsanteria.com/changoacute.html.

living human shamans, Indo-European or Scythian. In recent years, several tombs of Caucasian shamans were found in China, Mongolia, and other places far from the Central Asian mountains. The shamans, of course, had large amounts of cannabis buried with them. Perhaps one or more of these were responsible for the kernel of legend that became Indra.

In some traditions there is a distinction made between the ancestors whose names we can remember and the ones whose identities were lost through time. In voodoo, for instance, the unnamed ancestors are the barons and the ones we remember more accurately are the loas themselves, great human figures of history, and our more recently departed family members. Considering the suppressed history of cannabis, for many of us our higher ancestors may fall into the category of the unnamed.

RECALLING OUR FORGOTTEN ANCESTORS

Banish a space in which to work using expansion and contraction breathing or a banishing ritual of your choice. In that space, meditate or use self-hypnosis to enter a trance state. Get high by whatever means you find most agreeable. Then think about whatever you know about your genealogy, where your parents came from, their parents, your great-great-grandparents, etc. Think about the ancient people that your family arose from, how they may have lived, what kind of things they did to survive, live, and have fun. If you think there was a history of cannabis use, think about how they may have enjoyed their herb. Did they drink soma or bhang? Did they smoke it? Did they wear clothing made from hemp? Did they come from a culture that may have used hemp cloth as funeral clothing? Pay attention to how all this makes you feel.

Then welcome your ancestors: "Welcome, ancestors whose names have been forgotten!"

Make an offering to them, placing some cannabis or something else they may have valued on an altar. Burn some cannabis in an incense censer or in a pipe. Offer the smoke to the ancestors.

Offer your continued reverence to the ancestors and a promise to make more cannabis or other offerings. Then ask them to guide and protect you, to teach you, and to bring their wisdom into the present and future.

Sit quietly for a few minutes and notice whatever thoughts, feelings, images, etc. come to mind. Then thank the ancestors and close your ritual, reabsorbing anything you have imagined back into you.

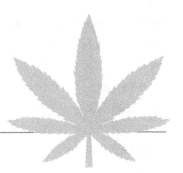

CHAPTER TWENTY-THREE
DIVINATION

Divination refers to a set of practices used to gain insight into a question or situation. In the more exoteric sense, we think of these methods as fortune-telling, although that doesn't really capture the varieties of experiences that result from divination. To pick on an obvious couple of methods, tarot cards or astrology are often used to provide fortune-cookie predictions of future events, but both those methods are also used as a way of contemplating and understanding how the individual psyche works and relates to the world. Fortune-telling can give some practice with the techniques and may begin the process of sorting consciousness into a balanced and well-integrated form, which is one of several long-term outcomes from divination.

Divination is one of those human experiences for which there is little scientific verification (or interest, for that matter) but which is reported from almost every culture on the planet. Indeed, there are so many different forms of divination that a complete list would take up many pages. To simplify things a bit, we can shuffle them into two main categories: trance techniques and holistic symbol systems. These two categories are not mutually exclusive; we also find many hybrid techniques that combine trance with symbols.

Holistic symbol systems include the tarot, I Ching, Ifa, geomancy, runes, and many more. In each of these, a collection of symbols represents a kind of cross section of reality. The complete set of symbols represents the world (as a microcosm) and the individual symbols represent each kind of experience we can have within that world. The total range of symbols in each system constitutes a holon, a representation of a whole, a simplified reflection of the universe.

Divination that relies on trance usually involves contemplating some natural phenomenon, a reflective surface of some kind, or a "random" pattern such as the residue in the bottom of a teacup, the entrails of a slain animal, or the ashes left from burning something. The practitioner enters a trance state, lets his or her mind go blank, and allows the shapes to suggest feelings, words, and images.

Many magicians who use symbol systems for divination will also employ trance techniques to help gain intuition from the symbols.

Historically, cannabis was important to many kinds of divination, more obviously in the trance category but also for drawing connections between symbols and for opening consciousness to a wider variety of possibilities.

In his treatise on the tarot, *The Book of Thoth*, Aleister Crowley includes a piece he wrote many years earlier, "Liber Aleph," that in a carefully clandestine manner, describes the method of using cannabis, "the Grass of the Arabs," for divination:

DE HERBO SANCTISSIMO ARABICO.

O my Son, yester Eve came the Spirit upon me that I also should eat the Grass of the Arabs, and by Virtue of the Bewitchment thereof behold that which might be appointed for the Enlightenment of mine Eyes. Now then of this may I not speak, seeing that it involveth the Mystery of the Transcending of Time, so that in One Hour of our terrestrial Measure did I gather the Harvest of an Aeon, and in Ten Lives I could not declare it.

DE QUIBUSDAM MYSTERIIS, QUAE VIDI.

Yet even as a Man may set up a Memorial or Symbol to import Ten Thousand Times Ten Thousand, so may I strive to inform thine Understanding by Hieroglyph ... Here first then is one amid the uncounted Wonders of that Vision; upon a field blacker and richer than Velvet was the Sun of all Being, alone. Then about Him were little Crosses, Greek,

over-running the Heaven. These changed from Form to Form geo-
metrical, Marvel devouring Marvel, a Thousand Times a Thousand in
their Course and Sequence, until by their Movement was the Universe
churned into the Quintessence of Light. Moreover at another Time did
I behold All Things as Bubbles, iridescent and luminous, self-shining in
every Colour, Myriad pursuing Myrad until by their perpetual Beauty
they exhausted the Virtue of my Mind to receive them, and whelmed
it, so that I was fain to withdraw myself from the Burden of that Bril-
liance. Yet, o my Son, the Sun of all this amounteth not to the Worth of
one Dawn-Glimmer of Our True Vision of Holiness.

DE QUORUM MODO MEDITATIONES.

Now for the Chief of that which was granted unto me, it was the Appre-
hension of those willed Changes or Transmutations of the Mind which
lead into Truth, being as Ladders unto Heaven, or so I called them at
that Time, seeking for a Phrase to admonish the Scribe that attended on
my Words, to grave a Balustre upon the Stele of of my Working. But I
make Effort in vain, o my Son, to record this matter in Detail; for it is
he quality of the Grass to quicken the Operation of Thought it may be
Thousandfold, and moreover to figure each Step in Images complex and
overpowering in Beauty, so that one hath no Time wherein to conceive,
much less to utter, any Word for a Name or any of them. Also, such
was the multiplicity of these Ladders, and their Equivalence, that the
Memory holdeth no more any one of them, but only a certain Compre-
hension of the Method, wordless by Reason of its Subtilty. Now therefore must I make by my Will a Concentration mighty and terrible of
my Thought, that I may bring forth this Mystery in Expression. For this
Method is of Virtue and Profit, by it mayst thou come easily and with
Delight to the Perfection of Truth, it is no Odds from what Thought
thou makest the first Leap in thy Meditation, so that thou mayst know
how every Road endeth in Monsalvat, and the Temple of the Sangral.[125]

---

125. Crowley, 1974.

Here Crowley gives a beautiful description of a cannabis experience including characteristic closed-eye hallucinations, time distortion, and transderivational search. While he declines to speak of it (due to either the nature of the revelation or the difficultly inherent in describing such altered states), we can infer that he derived his unspeakable knowledge, wisdom, or information from a free association based on the panoply of thoughts and patterns of the vision.

His method is similar to and probably influenced by the clairvoyance techniques described by P. B. Randolph, who studied with the mesmerists in France. Randolph used a broad definition of clairvoyance and described a variety of specific techniques. Under the general heading of clairvoyance, Randolph included clairvoyance, in which the magician in trance sees the information being sought; psychometry, in which contact with a person or object stimulates feelings in the magician, which are interpreted to yield information; and intuition, in which answers come into consciousness and are tested by the magician.[126]

Randolph described the somewhat overly complicated techniques of mesmerism as a means to enter trance and conduct this kind of divination. He then suggested that the practitioner use a pool of ink or a mirror as a scrying tool, something to gaze into while you allow a vision to come. In separate writings, he also described a much simpler method of inducing trance: hashish.[127]

Where a person takes hashish for any purpose, let that purpose be clearly, firmly, solidly fixed in the mind from the moment the drug is taken till its effect is over. For instance, if it be to become clairvoyant, let that, and no other object be sought for. If to be a speaker, medium, to find absent persons, property, to know the state of a love that's doubted; to find if a love is true or false; if one is pregnant, or anything else (and there are few problems that cannot be solved, under hashish), let that one object, and no other, engage attention. This being resolved upon, when the clairvoyance bursts upon you, as it probably will, give the

---

126. Randolph, P. B. *Seership! The Magnetic Mirror: A Practical Guide for Those Who Aspire to Clairvoyance.* Forgotten Books, 2018.

127. Bennett, 2018.

whole soul to the matter in hand, and as soon as the reply is had, instantly break the spell as above directed.[128]

Randolph also recommended infrequent use, suggesting that once clairvoyance was made possible through the use of hashish, it would always be possible again, with or without cannabis.

The central technique used in Randolph's clairvoyance and in many other trance techniques is known as scrying. Scrying is the practice of staring into a visually ambiguous medium and allowing the mind to free associate from the shapes and images seen within. The well-known practice of fortune-telling by gazing into a crystal ball is a form of scrying. Along with crystals, bowls of water, pools of ink, mirrors of various sorts, clouds, landscapes, stones, fire, and smoke are often employed. One of my own favorite methods is to sit on the bank of a river and watch the interplay of wind and light on the surface of the water.

BASIC SCRYING

Establish a light trance state as you best know how. Gaze into the medium of your choice. If you have a particular question or subject about which you hope to gain insight, frame that question in your mind as you gaze. As the shapes you see within the medium or in your own mind begin to appear, state them out loud. Think of this first stage as being like cloud-watching. What do the random shapes or images suggest to your mind? Continue this process, allowing your trance state to deepen and the complexity of the images to increase. Be patient and allow the images to begin to suggest people, places, objects, and stories.

BASIC PSYCHOMETRY

Choose an object or person about which you would like to gain insight. Enter a light trance as best you can. Hold the object or touch the person (in a mutually agreed upon way). Focus your attention on the feeling of the object or

---

128. Randolph, P. B. "Hashish. Its Uses, Abuses, and Dangers, Its Extasia, Fantasia, and Illuminati." (1867). Published in "The Hidden Hash Master of the 19th Century: Paschal Beverly Randolph" by Chris Bennett, *Cannabis Culture,* November 2016.

person. As you allow the feeling to fill your awareness, notice whatever other feelings arise in your body. Allow whatever thoughts may be associated with those feelings to come into your mind. For instance, a feeling in the pit of the stomach may suggest loss or sadness (or almost anything else; these associations are mostly personal). Feelings may suggest love, happiness, sensuality, anger, sadness, detachment, compassion, yearning, excitement, revelation, or any other emotional or visceral experience. Allow the complexity of the feelings to build. If the feelings are accompanied by visions, sounds, or words, welcome them, note what they are, and return to your awareness of the feelings.

With practice, the insights from scrying and psychometry can come quicker and with more detail. As an initial exploration, you can follow the general pattern we've been using for many of the exercises in this book: practice both without and with cannabis.

There are a few specifically cannabis-derived scrying mediums that can be explored easily. You can gaze at leaves (phyllomancy) either still on the plant or piled randomly in a large bowl. Sometimes a little movement, the wind through the leaves of a field of hemp for instance, can give more depth and associations to the medium. Even the patterns of crystalline resin glands on a bud can inspire a kind of phyllomancy. Gazing at the shapes found in smoke (turifumy), or the patterns found in ashes (cineromancy) are also useful methods.

Cannabis also provides us with a very unique and effective scrying medium: your own eyelids. A good dose of cannabis, especially with a high-THC strain, can produce closed-eye visuals, including shifting clouds of color, sparkling lights, swirling geometrics, lattice patterns, faces, cartoon images, landscapes, and so on. These can be observed and used as the seed for free association, just as you might give attention to the shapes in a crystal or clouds. Combining cannabis with a trance technique can intensify the visuals and the associations derived from them.

Holistic symbol systems provide more information up front, as it were, by attaching a meaning to each symbol and a randomizing method to select each one. The challenge to the magician is interpreting the symbols in context. For instance, one may shuffle a deck of tarot cards and draw three of them (or more, of course) for a reading. The symbols on the cards are necessarily vague—they suggest patterns in the world rather than every specific possibility that can occur. It is the reader's job to apply them to the person and situation at hand. This requires the ability to draw connections between the symbols and to fit them into a narrative, a story that reveals something about the querent. In terms of brain functions, once again we are seeing an interplay between executive function and the narrative-generating imagination of the default network.

Crowley's inclusion of the "Liber Aleph" essay concerning the "Sacred Grass of the Arabs" in his treatise on tarot, *The Book of Thoth*, was a slightly veiled but otherwise unambiguous endorsement of cannabis as an aid to this kind of divination.

The techniques that I consider hybrids are mostly derived by attempts to codify the more random types of scrying. That is, over time, when patterns are repeated in similar circumstances, a magician may start to recognize those patterns and correlations and list them in ways that can be passed along to others. In this way, we get books that show patterns in bottoms of teacups, interpretations of the lines on someone's hand, and so on. Some of the more well-known symbol systems may have begun in this way. For instance, the I Ching had its origin in observations of tossed yarrow stalks[129] or the markings on a tortoise's shell. Even the patterns and colors of closed-eye visuals may be codified in this way. P. B. Randolph attributed meaning to the colors of "clouds" that he saw when mirror-gazing:

> White clouds are favorable; affirmative; good … Black clouds are the exact reverse: inauspicious; bad … Violet, green, blue, presage coming joy—are excellent … Red, crimson, orange, yellow, mean danger, trouble, sickness, "beware," deceptions, losses, betrayal, slander, grief, and indicate surprises of a disagreeable character.[130]

---

129. Also hemp stalks.
130. Randolph, 2018.

There are numerous books about tarot, I Ching, and other symbol-based divination methods.[131] While a magician can continue to deepen his or her knowledge of any one of these systems over a lifetime, the basic techniques are usually pretty simple and can be learned in a few days. Again, I'll offer the general method: practice and learn the methods without cannabis first, then notice how it differs when you add some ganja to your consciousness.

---

131. See the Suggested Reading section toward the end of this book.

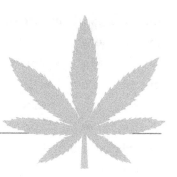

CHAPTER TWENTY-FOUR
HIGH MAGICK

Some practitioners make a distinction between practical (or low) magick and high magick. In short, practical magick is about doing stuff in the world—finding relationships, gaining wealth, developing health, countering enemies or adversity, and so on. High magick, on the other hand, is about what we might call personal development, traditionally with the aid of a deity or pantheon. The idea is that you can make yourself a better person first, deepening your understanding of the world in a way, gaining wisdom that makes practical decisions and plans easier to arrive at. One way of understanding high magick is that we use ritual techniques to align ourselves with the universe (or deity) in such a way that our lives become more meaningful, effective, and, hopefully, happier.

Eliphas Levi, a famous occultist of the nineteenth century, described the Great Work as "…the creation of man by himself, that is to say, the full and entire conquest of his faculties and his future; it is especially the perfect emancipation of his will."[132] Aleister Crowley concurred with Levi, and also suggested that the method of the Great Work included the "union of opposites," which he explained by saying, "It may mean the uniting of the soul with God, of the

---

132. Levi, Eliphas. *Transcendental Magic: Its Doctrine and Ritual.* Martino Fine Books, 2011.

microcosm with the macrocosm, of the female with the male, of the ego with the non-ego."[133]

In Crowley's system, the new initiate would concentrate solely on learning about true will, his or her proper course through the universe. With a nod to astrophysics, Crowley expressed this with the statement "Every man and woman is a star," suggesting that we each have our own natural path in the metaphoric galaxy of our lives. The vector of the star is not something easily named, however, and while our overall course through life may describe a continuous arc, the specifics of true will at each moment may change. That is to say, we are not easily defined by our jobs, our careers, or our accomplishments, and even a superhero or a saint has to make breakfast or go to the toilet every now and then.

Crowley's system, known as Thelema,[134] includes a body of ritual aimed at discovering and attaining true will. When guided by true will, the magician can then practice magick intended to change the world either on a personal level or a societal one.

The broadest idea of high magick—that we can improve ourselves and thereby make better decisions about our lives—remains useful, although sometimes there's a big overlap between self-improvement and survival (or self-enrichment, for that matter). As mentioned in an earlier chapter, schools of high magick tend to be systematic, guiding the aspirant through invocations and evocations that represent, once again, a holon, all the spheres, all the elements, all the ranks of entities available. In this way, the magician becomes well-rounded, complete, a human with a full range of resources, skills, and experiences.[135]

At the simplest end of high magick, a basic act of ritual framing can change the context of an experience and can open the way to more complex practice. A good example of this is the prayer that many say before meals. In the main-

---

133. Crowley, Aleister. *Magick Without Tears*. 8th Printing Edition. New Falcon, 1991.
134. Greek for "Will."
135. An old magick joke goes like this: Q: What do you call a magician who specializes in the element of fire? A: Unbalanced.

stream context, that prayer is "grace," a thank-you to the deity. Grace reminds Christians and others who might practice it that their lives are intimately connected with their deity and that whatever they have, no matter how meager or abundant, is a gift from their creator. In a magical context, that ritual might be "Saying Will," as Crowley proposed it:

1: Do what thou wilt shall be the whole of the Law.

2: What is our Will?

3: It is our Will to eat and drink.

4: For what purpose?

5: That we may continue to do the Great Work.

6: What is the Great Work?

7: [Gives brief statement about current work, i.e., "It is my Will to continue writing a book."]

8: Love is the Law, Love under Will.[136]

"Saying Will" is a simple ritual frame and it may be easy to see how it can be adapted for a cannabis session:

1: Do what thou wilt shall be the whole of the Law.

2: What is our Will?

3: It is our Will to [smoke, vape, ingest] our magick herb.

4: For what purpose?

Etc.

Note the similarity of this practice to the toasting or framing rituals used by sadhus, Rastas, and others. A sadhu will praise Shiva before using the chillum and a Rasta will offer praise to Jah Rastafari or thanks to Jah for the herb.

---

136. Crowley, Aleister. *Magick: Book 4*, second edition. York Beach, ME: Samuel Weiser, 1997.

WAKE-N-BAKE FRAMES

Wake-n-Bake is a common ritual among cannabis enthusiasts and medical patients. Very simply, it involves having a few tokes upon waking.[137] It's an act that sets the tone for the day, and by applying a little conscious ritualizing, it's possible to influence that daily tone in a variety of ways.

1. Visualize an image of yourself, sitting or standing in front of you.

2. Modify that image until it represents the you that you'd like to experience during the day. Pay attention to the image's posture, breathing, facial expression, and what it may be doing with its hands.

3. If there is a particular activity for the day that you know you'll be involved with (going to work, driving your car, creating art, socializing, etc.), see the image of yourself engaged in that activity with joy, passion, skill, or whatever qualities you choose. If you don't know what you'll be doing during the day, eliminate background and context, keeping a joyful, passionate, skillful (or whatever) image of yourself.

4. If there are any sounds associated with this image, imagine hearing them.

5. Take a moment and contemplate the image. Notice any feelings you may have while looking at it.

6. Take a toke, inhaling that image. Imagine the energy of the image filling you from head to toe.

7. Allow that energy to push out any remnants of sleep and any thoughts, feelings, etc. that are contrary to your plans for the day. Exhale those remnants.

8. Finish your wake-n-bake and go about your day.

TOASTING AND PRAISING

A toast is one of the simplest forms of ritual frame, but as we've seen, even simple ritual frames can be effective. Everyone has done it at one point or an-

---

137. The downside to wake-n-bake is that daily use and morning use can increase your tolerance to cannabis significantly. In other words, if you want to get high later in the day, you'll need to consume a greater amount.

other, usually with alcoholic beverages. "To your health!" or some variant of that is the most common. More complex beverage toasts are composed for special events, awards, weddings, and so on, where the participants are praised and toasted.

Cannabis toasts are more often (these days, at any rate) found in a religious context. Shivites will praise Shiva before inhaling or drinking their cannabis. Rastas will praise Haile Selassie or give thanks to Jah before smoking a spliff.

So what is it that you want to toast? Whom do you wish to praise?

Toast Examples

Health, wealth, and happiness!

To your health!

Peace!

Infinite harmony!

To the project at hand!

Creativity!

May you find joy in all you do!

Happy holiday!

Praise Examples

Ma Gu brings good fortune!

Boom boom Mahadev! (Hail great god, Shiva!)

To the spirit of the plant!

Jah Rastafari!

To my wonderful friends!

To my future self!

THE TALKING JOINT

The talking joint is the cannabis counterpart of the talking stick in Native American tradition (along with very similar traditions in Africa and other parts of the world). The talking stick is usually a carved wooden staff that is passed around during group meetings. As a way to keep order during gatherings, while the stick makes its rounds, only the person who is presently holding it may speak. The method may also be used to create a consensus-based ritual frame in which everyone has a chance to be included. It is a good way to get everyone involved in a project and as a way to start group meetings of any kind.

THE TALKING JOINT

1. Roll a special, large joint for your group or employ a ceremonial pipe that is used specifically and only for this purpose. The joint or bowl should be large enough to be passed around to everyone present at least once.

2. The group assembles in a circle and it is decided which way the joint will pass and if there is a particular purpose or theme.

3. As each person receives the joint, he or she makes a short statement of what they would like to accomplish with their altered state. This can be a simple toast or a statement of intent.

4. After making the statement, he or she takes a toke and exhales their intent into the center of the circle.

5. He or she passes the joint to the next person.

6. When the joint has been passed to everyone present and each person has made a statement (or silence if they choose), the joint can either continue its rounds until finished (without statements), or it can come in for a landing in an ashtray.

7. The meeting, project, or party can commence.

SMOKE OF EXCELLENCE

The Circle of Excellence is a classic NLP exercise to demonstrate anchoring, the intentional use of conditioned experience to reaccess useful and enjoyable states.[138] With a few modifications for simplicity, it can become a cannabis magick technique.

---

138. Dilts, Robert, and Judith DeLozier. *Encyclopedia of of Systemic Neuro-Linguistic Programming and NLP New Coding.* NLP University Press, 2000.

Smoke of Excellence

1. Think of a pleasant, useful, or peak experience that you've had recently or in the past that you would like to reexperience.

2. Imagine a circle on the floor. Stand just outside the circle, facing it. Have a joint or bowl ready to light.

3. Begin to remember the experience. Remember what you saw at that time, if there was movement or stillness in your field of vision. Notice what the colors were like and if it was brightly lit or dim. As you remember what you saw, recall what you heard at that time, sounds or silence, voices, tones, rhythms, and background sounds. And as you continue to remember what you saw and heard, remember how you felt, the position of your body, any movements you may have made, the temperature of the air on your skin, and anything that you may have been in contact with.

4. As you recall the memory, remember what the experience of the desired state itself felt like, where in your body you could feel it, and what kind of feeling it was (temperature, pressure, tingling, movement, texture, or whatever it may have been).

5. If that feeling had a color or colors, what would it be? Apply the color everywhere in your body that you have the feeling.

6. Take a deep toke. As you exhale, imagine that you send the color from your feeling along with the smoke into the circle, creating an imagined column of color.

7. Repeat steps 1 through 6.

8. Shake off the state, take a deep breath, let it go.

9. Step into the circle and notice how much of the state returns.

10. Repeat steps 1 through 9 as necessary to increase the power of the state.

11. Step out of the circle and imagine that you are picking the circle up from the floor, rolling it up, and placing it in your pocket or another safe place.

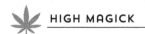

12. At another time when you'd like to reaccess the state, take out the circle, place it on the floor, step in.

GROUP CHARGING

This is a kind of banishing/charging ritual for two or more participants (the more the merrier!) to prepare a space, an object, or consumables for group use.

Group Charging

1. Sit in a circle (or facing each other, if it's only two people) with the object to be charged in the center. If you are preparing a space, sit evenly spaced around the circumference of the area, facing the space to be charged.

2. Decide on the quality that you wish to share during the meeting or when using the object/consumables. For instance, if your meeting is to create something together, the quality might be creativity or ingenuity. If the intent is to socialize, the quality might be fun or intimacy.

3. A joint or bowl is prepared. If participants are sitting too far away from each other to easily pass a joint (when charging a space), then each can have their own joint or bowl.

4. Each participant recalls or imagines a situation in which they experienced the quality that was decided upon.

5. As in the previous exercise, each person remembers what they saw at that time, if there was movement or stillness in their field of vision. Notice what the colors were like and if it was brightly lit or dim. As each person remembers what they saw, they can recall what was heard at that time, sounds or silence, voices, tones, rhythms, and background sounds. And as they continue to remember what was seen and heard, they can remember how it felt, the position of their body, any movements that may have been made, the temperature of the air on skin, and anything that they may have been in contact with.

6. As each person recalls the memory, they can remember what the experience of the desired state itself felt like, where in their body they could

feel it, and what kind of feeling it was (temperature, pressure, tingling, movement, texture, or whatever it may have been).

7. If that feeling had a color or colors, what would they be? Each person applies the color everywhere in their body where they have the feeling.

8. In turn or simultaneously, each participant takes a deep toke. As each person exhales, they imagine sending the color along with the smoke into the space or object.

9. When each person has completed this, the space can then be used for the meeting or project, the object can be employed in whatever way was intended, or the consumables can be shared among everyone. Note what it feels like or what thoughts come to mind as you use the space, object, or consumables.

Cannabis enters Western esoteric traditions in two primary ways. First, as already discussed at some length, getting high helps establish a useful state of mind that encourages possibility, focus on the present, and the use of imagination. As a ritual enhancer, cannabis helps with the processes of magick, no matter what quality, sphere, deity, or entity you are working with. And cannabis can, itself, be categorized qabalistically, becoming one element, one quality to explore among all the elements and qualities in the world that can be explored. Crowley's classification of cannabis as a Eucharist of three elements falls more sqaurely into the first category, something that can be used in a wide range of ritual and exploration.

To find the specific qualities of cannabis in the systems of magick, we can turn to Crowley's lengthy lists of qabalistic correspondences, *777*, where he lists cannabis as "Indian Hemp" and attributes the plant to the Twenty-Sixth Path of the Tree of Life, which corresponds to the tarot card the Devil,[139] the Greek god Pan, the Egyptian Set, the Hebrew letter Ayin (which means "an eye"), and the secret title of "The Lord of the Gates of Matter, The Child of

---

139. When Christianity supplanted local Pagan traditions in Europe, the old horned nature deities were branded as demons as a way to discredit and draw followers from the native religions. Pan himself became the Devil and depictions of the Christian adversary took on Pan's goat-like appearance.

the Forces of Time."[140] Robert Wang, in his giant treatise on the tarot, *Qabalistic Tarot*, ascribes to the Twenty-Sixth Path the even more secret—and very fitting—quality of "Mirth."[141]

The Twenty-Sixth Path runs between Tiphareth (Sphere #6) and Hod (Sphere #8) on the Tree of Life. To fully fathom the meanings of such qabalistic concepts takes years—maybe a lifetime—of study. The study itself can be considered high magick as it is a way of ordering the elements of consciousness into a kind of mental filing cabinet that lets us know which drawers still need to be filled, cleaned, or otherwise given attention. It can be used as a kind of blueprint for structuring the mind of the magician. With that said, the quick take is that Tiphareth is the very center of being itself, symbolized by the sun and corresponding to such things as beauty, glory, and true will. Hod is the sphere of science, language, and thought, Hermes, Mercury, and Thoth. As Lord of the Gates of Matter, the Twenty-Sixth Path represents, in a sense, how we create our reality from thoughts, models, beliefs, and words. As the tarot Devil card, the path suggests that we are, in a sense, tied to matter and imprisoned by our models and beliefs. We come to mistake those models for absolute external reality, rather than a product of our consciousness. As the path runs both ways, cannabis plays a role in reality selection—and also in dishabituation, the variety of consciousness that frees us from dogma and conditioning.

So when we explore the entities found on this path, it's not surprising that they are tricksters. The spirits of the Twenty-Sixth Path appear through history, variously, as Pan, the goat-footed Greek god of fertility, creativity, and panic; as the medieval hobgoblin Robin Goodfellow; as the Green Man; and as the Sufi hash-spirit Khidr. In Crowley's system, the Twenty-Sixth Path represented (among other things) "Creativity without lust of result," the experience of being fully engaged in your art, in the moment, enjoying the process.

The technique of exploring a path on the Tree of Life is called pathworking. In general, pathworking involves entering a trance state in which the path

---

140. Crowley, Aleister. *777 and Other Qabalistic Writings.* Weiser Books, 1986.

141. Wang, Robert. *The Qabalistic Tarot.* U.S. Games Systems, 2017.

is explored as if it were a realm of its own, a place in which each perception reflects, in some way, the qualities of the path.

PATHWORKING THE TWENTY-SIXTH PATH (OR ANY OTHER ONE)

Obtain a tarot card that relates to the qabalistic path that you wish to explore. In this case, the Twenty-Sixth Path, the Devil card can be used. The cards in different decks created by different authors will each depict different aspects of the path. Choose a card from a deck that appeals to you, about which you feel some kind of resonance and comfort with the style of the artwork. Place the card on an altar in front of you. Enter a trance by whatever means you know best. (For the Twenty-Sixth Path, some cannabis may be used along with a hypnotic or meditative technique.) Gaze at the card and remember the image on it so that when you close your eyes you can still (imagine that you) see it. In your mind's eye, allow the image of the card to grow larger, to the size of a door... and let it become a door; open it and go through the doorway.

Once through, take a look down at your (astral, imagined) feet. Notice the ground (or whatever it is you're standing on) next to your feet. Then allow your gaze to move outward, including more ground, and whatever else is in the sphere of your attention. Explore this realm as best you can. When you are finished, reabsorb all your imaginings, open your eyes, and write down or record your thoughts about what you experienced in the astral realm.

To practice the systematic exploration of *all* the spheres, paths, elements, planets, signs, etc. (depending on what system you prefer), along with pathworking and other techniques, we have three basic operations: banishing, invocation, and evocation. In general, we think of banishing as the rituals and methods that we use to clear out a space prior to working, sort of like a psychic broom that chases away the dust bunnies of distraction. It's not quite that simple, though. Much like when we meditate, if we clear something away (or repress it or try not to think about it), we leave a void that is quickly filled by other thoughts. The trick with many so-called banishing rituals is that they are also invocations and evocations, too. That is, they don't create a psychic vacuum, they banish unwanted qualities and thoughts by filling the circle with your own aura or energy or the energy of evoked entities.

We've already used one technique as an extremely simple banishing: expansion and contraction breathing, which uses your own breath and energy to fill and banish an area. More complex but popular banishings include rituals such as the Lesser Banishing Ritual of the Pentagram, the Star Ruby, and others. These are often presented to new magicians as the first rituals to be studied and practiced as they not only prepare the ritual space and consciousness of the practitioner but also teach basic techniques. These rituals are widely available in books on magick and on the internet, so I won't repeat them here. It is also very helpful to learn and practice them, if you can, with someone who is experienced with the methods. Simply hearing how the words are pronounced and vibrated and experiencing the feeling of a successfully completed banishing can be an important step toward mastery.

Invocation is the practice of drawing qualities or entities into our consciousness. While that may sound particularly magical, we often engage in similar behaviors without considering them to be occult. If you have a song that inspires you that you listen to before working or playing, for instance, that's a form of invocation. If you've ever gone into a church or temple, looked at the artwork and iconography, and been moved in some way, that's invocation. If you've ever written or recited a poem about a person or entity and felt excited, enthused, or otherwise emotional, you've experienced a form of invocation. In a system of high magick, the rituals may include elements of all of the above—imagery, music, poetry, and more—for the purpose of exploring and engaging with the entire range of a pantheon, all the elements of a system, or however the various qualities are categorized.

Evocation is when we relate to a quality or entity as if it is external to us. So, when you were a kid (or more recently!) and you spoke or played with your imaginary friend, you were performing evocation. If you've ever written fiction and created a character that you put in a story, that's a form of evocation. In the more traditional magical context, evocation takes the form of summoning spirits, contacting various entities, and communicating with them.

The set of elements to be explored in every system, ideally, can be thought of as a holon, as a microcosmic reflection of the whole world in which we live. The complexity of a system depends on the number of pieces we are willing to divide the universe into. At the simple end, we have systems of two elements: yin and yang. There are systems of four elements: fire, water, air, and earth. Or five elements, seven planets, eight circuits, ten Sephirah, twelve signs of the zodiac, sixty-four hexagrams of the I Ching, and so on. In the spirit of creating microcosms, here's a possible cannabis holon and ritual.

CANNABIS MAGICK HOLON RITUAL

Soil—the basis, the raw materials, the ancestors

Air—purification, catalysis, the elements that stoke the fire

Sun—energy, will, fire, power to do things

Roots—stability, transformation (of soil to nutrients), connections to others

Stalk—strength, support, transport (of nutrients to cells)

Leaves—interface with environment, transformation (of sun to growth)

Flowers—culmination, harvest, thoughts, ideas, beauty, inspiration

Smoke—transformation, death, aspiration, transience

Seed—potential, start of a new cycle, thoughts of the future

As with most "holonic" categories, these provide a sort of mental filing cabinet in which to sort and classify thoughts, things, and experiences. Taken together, the categories describe the process of growth, how plants, people, poems, politics, and many other things come about, from the raw materials to the harvest.

WEEK ONE

1. As you go through your days, notice each thing that makes you think about soil, in both literal and metaphoric ways. What are the fertile raw materials of your life? In what do you plant the seeds of your ideas? Write down the ones that seem like the strongest impressions or the most important.

2. On the seventh day of your soil week, perform the following ritual:

    a. Banish with the method of your choice.

    b. Sit and meditate in the space for a few minutes.

    c. Recall the various soil-related experiences you had during the week, including the ones you have written down.

    d. Smoke (or otherwise use your cannabis) and allow your mind to spin off ideas, images, sounds, words, feelings, or whatever kind of transderivational search your soil-related thoughts inspire.

    e. As you notice these thoughts and perceptions, allow them to flow into a ball of energy that you imagine in front of you within the banished space.

    f. Toke and breathe into the ball of energy, notice what it does in your mind's eye. Notice if it has a color, a shape, motion, or any other defining characteristics. Does the shape or color make you think of something?

    g. Take another toke; as you exhale intone the word "soil."

    h. Handle the ball of energy. Notice what it feels like in your hands. Place it back within you. Notice how that feels or what thoughts it might inspire.

    i. Write down what you've learned about the soil ball of energy, about soil in general, and anything else of interest.

WEEKS TWO THROUGH NINE

1. Perform the same practices for each of the other qualities: air, sun, roots, stalk, leaves, flowers, smoke, seed.

FINALE

1. Banish with the method of your choice.

2. Sit and meditate for a few minutes.

3. Reestablish each energy ball by intoning the word ("soil," "air," etc.) and imagining the ball's color, size, shape, etc.

4. Arrange the balls at the tips of imaginary leaflets with you sitting in the center of the leaf where all the leaflets join.

5. Toke and breathe into each energy ball.

6. Notice how it feels and what thoughts are in your mind.

7. Draw all the energy balls together into one large ball just in front of you. Notice what it does, what colors it takes, what shape, etc. Breathe into it and notice what it does.

8. Bring the combined energy ball into you. Allow it to flow through your body, to all the parts of you that it is willing to go. Notice how this feels and what thoughts are in your mind.

9. If you wish, smoke for a few minutes and enjoy the experience.

10. Banish again, clearing the space and reabsorbing any imaginings still external to you. Keep however much of the feeling and thoughts from the ritual as you deem appropriate.

As with most high magick, this ritual is (mostly) not used for a stated practical purpose (though there are ways it can be adapted for such use). Rather, the idea of the ritual is to fill, balance, and realign your consciousness. Various thoughts and ideas may occur to you as you practice this ritual. Record them in whatever way is best for you.

The ritual work in some traditions increases in complexity as the magician continues through the system. For some people, this kind of complexity works well as a way of overloading the conscious mind so that unconscious factors can go to work.[142] For others, simplicity is the key. Which you choose may depend on your existing tendencies and your goals for the future. My suggestion is to start at the simple end of things and if you develop curiosity about the structure and use of more intense rituals, then keep on going. If you start exploring a system, though, commit to following it through.

---

142. Indeed, some writers consider occult qabala to be a kind of joke that gets us to transcend our usual consciousness, comparable to a Zen koan in use and effect but infinitely more complex.

The Cannabis Magick Holon ritual is extremely simple as high magick systems go. With this, I'm mostly hoping to provide a basis for more involved work and to offer a glimpse into the nature and structure of magick in general. If you are interested in delving deeper into the ideas of traditional high magick systems, see the Suggested Reading section at the end of the book.

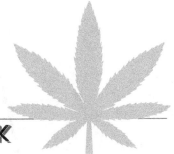

CHAPTER TWENTY-FIVE
PRACTICAL MAGICK

There are numerous methods of practical magick, the art of making things happen and getting things done. Each of us will have preferences and techniques that work better than others, for us. Here are three examples of techniques that can be easily adapted to cannabis magick.

SIGILS

Sigils are simple (or not so simple) drawings that encapsulate and symbolize a more complex outcome or goal. The sigil itself is a kind of anchor that connects your present experience to a state, a behavior, or an outcome. There are a variety of different ways to generate sigils, discussed at length in other books on magick or easily found on the internet. Two simple methods are included here and if you know or prefer other methods, use the one you feel most comfortable with.

Smokin' Sigils

1. Sigil Method #1: Write out a short statement of what you will create a sigil to accomplish. For instance, "Making Money." Then eliminate vowels: *M, K, N, G,* and *M, N, Y.* Then eliminate any duplicate letters: *M, K, N, G, Y.* Then be creative and combine the letters into a single symbol. An easy and simplified version is on the top, and a more stylized version is on the bottom. Be as creative as you can.

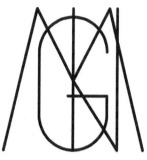

Simple Version

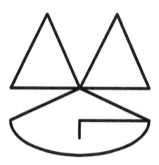

Stylized Version

2. Sigil Method #2 (If you don't like playing with letters): Think about how it will feel to have the outcome you desire. For instance, if your outcome is making money, imagine holding a check for a large sum, seeing amounts accruing in your bank balance, or however you choose to imagine it, and notice how this feels. Notice wherever you have that feeling in your body and give it a color or colors, as in previous exercises. Take a good look in your mind at that shape in your body and sketch the general outlines on paper. That sketch, representing the feeling in your body, can be used in place of a letter sigil.

3. Place the drawn sigil or sketch on your altar (or, generally, in front of you). Take a big toke and exhale the smoke into the sigil, imagining it absorbing the energy of your breath and becoming charged by it.

SMOKING SIGILS

1. Create a sigil. If you'd like, you can create it initially on a piece of rolling paper or, once created, redraw it on rolling paper and charge it in whatever way you find useful.

2. Roll a joint with the sigilized paper.

3. Smoke the joint, releasing the intent and outcome to the universe in the smoke that you exhale and the smoke that rises from the end of the joint.

4. Notice, over the next day or so, indications that your outcome has been accepted by the universe.

ENLISTING THE PLANT SPIRIT

In a few magical systems, manifestation magick is accomplished through an intermediary entity. In effect, we're already working via the cannabis plant spirit in most of these exercises, though we can do it more directly and consciously.

Plant Spirit Manifestation

1. Decide on an outcome, what you would like to have happen. This can be almost anything, although it is often more effective if you can imagine what the path to that outcome may be. That is, you can decide to make money, but it is more effective to include how you will make money and whatever actions or steps you will take. It is also helpful to frame the outcome as a positive. That is, instead of what you don't want ("I don't want to be hungry"), you can delineate what you do want ("I want an excellent meal in a good restaurant").

2. Create a space to work in and banish.

3. Contact the cannabis plant spirit using the method described in the chapter on entities.

4. Breath into the entity and ask if it will help you manifest your outcome. If the answer is yes, continue on. If the answer is no, ask what is necessary for the entity to help you. Fulfill those requirements if they are agreeable to you.

5. Imagine as many details of your outcome as you can. See it, hear it, feel it, taste it, smell it. As you imagine each detail, give it to the plant spirit.

6. Breathe into the entity and ask it to release the details of your outcome to all the parts of the universe necessary and appropriate to make it manifest as you've imagined it.

7. Observe as the entity releases the details to the universe. Notice any changes in the entity and any feelings that you may have.

8. Ask the entity if the outcome has been accepted by the universe. If yes, continue; if no, ask what will be necessary for it to be accepted.

9. Ask the entity to thank the universe for you. Then thank the entity.

10. Reabsorb the entity and any imaginings still external to you.

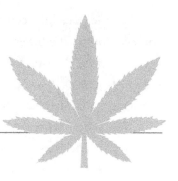

CHAPTER TWENTY-SIX

THE NEOSOMA
RITUAL

The Neosoma Ritual is an attempt to create a modern ceremony that fills the celebratory and mind-expanding place of the ancient soma and haoma rituals. This ritual pulls together a few of the major themes that we've explored and practiced so far in this book: framing, banishing, invocation, breathing, and the Cannabis Magick Holon among them. The Neosoma Ritual can be used for a variety of purposes; mainly, though, we use it as a means to connect with and become inspired by our deities and highest aspirations.

CONSECRATING THE SOMA

In ancient times, the essential bit of religion, spread by the Indo-Europeans and the Scythians, involved the soma sacrament. While archaeological evidence suggests that soma was most often cannabis, different plants were used in different places and times, based on local availability and customs. We also find that, in India when the preferred gods shifted from Indra to Shiva, soma was forbidden to all but the priests. However, bhang, essentially the same thing, was still widely used. So the question is…what was the difference between bhang and soma? What makes the particular plant or potion soma? The answer: magick.

The difference between bhang and soma was undoubtedly the ritual, the consecration of the beverage rather than the drink alone. A particular plant could fill in for the original soma plant because of the ritual. We don't know the exact ritual that was used in ancient times, although we have at least two surviving traditions that offer clues. The first of these is the Zoroastrian Ab-Zohr rite, the modern version of the ancient haoma ritual. The second is the Roman Catholic Mass, a survival of the soma/haoma rite via Mithraism.

In the Ab-Zohr rite, the haoma is consecrated through a lengthy process while the beverage is being prepared. The juice of the plant is expressed into milk at certain propitious times while invocations are recited. The Catholic Mass includes a series of prayers and offerings called the Anaphora, during which the bread and wine are transmuted into the body and blood of Christ. The climax of it is the Epiclesis, when the Holy Spirit is called down into the wine and wafers.

As magicians rather than necessarily religious adherents, we get some choice about the deity that we imbibe with our soma and there are several ways to make that decision. First, if there is a deity already known to you that you have worked with before and have some sense that it would be appropriate, you can consecrate your cannabis to that deity. You can work with a cannabis plant spirit. Or you can use meta-magical methods to access an entity that represents your highest aspirations. Recipes for bhang can be found on page 10 or use your own favorite method to produce a cannabis beverage.

CONSECRATION TO A KNOWN DEITY

1. Have a bowl or chalice that is used only for consecrating or holding consecrated cannabis. Prepare a fresh batch of bhang to be consecrated and put it in the special chalice.

2. Gather together images, songs, words, stories, etc. that relate to the deity that you choose. Place these in your working area.

3. Banish your space using a ritual or technique that you are familiar with. (For example, a simple banishing can be done with expansion and contraction breathing.)

4. Place the chalice of freshly made bhang on your altar or on the ground in front of you (if you don't have an actual altar).

5. Create an experience for yourself (and participants) of the deity. Display and study the images, sing the songs, recite the poems, tell the story of the deity.

6. Notice the unique feelings that are associated with this deity. Allow that feeling to build within you. If it helps to visualize, give it a color or colors.

7. Take a deep breath and, as you exhale, send that feeling and color along with whatever other thoughts and perceptions you have concerning the deity into the chalice of bhang. Say out loud, "I consecrate the contents of this chalice to [name of deity]."

8. Cover the chalice, wrap it in a piece of clean cloth (hemp if available), and place it in a special place until it is time to use it in ritual (soon, of course, while the milk is still good). The contents of the chalice are now considered soma.

CONSECRATION TO YOUR
HIGHEST ASPIRATION ENTITY

1. Have a bowl or chalice that is used only for consecrating or holding consecrated cannabis. Prepare a fresh batch of bhang to be consecrated and put it in the special chalice.

2. Banish your space using a ritual or technique familiar to you. (For example, a simple banishing can be done with expansion and contraction breathing.)

3. Think about what experiences and factors may relate to your highest aspirations in life. What times have you been closest to those aspirations? What would it feel like to have them? If you can't think of specific experiences or behaviors, be general and think about who you might be in an ideal world. What are the general results that might be expected? Happiness? Compassion? Equanimity? Or...?

4. Imagine that you see yourself, standing or sitting. Eliminate background noise and any accessories, objects, props, and so on that might be in your image so that the image is just you.

5. Begin to adjust the physiology of the imagined person to express more and more of your highest aspiration. Pay attention to and adjust facial expression, posture, breathing, movements, skin tone, muscle usage, and anything else that might pertain.

6. Adjust the structure of the image (submodalities) for greater impact. Experiment with image size, color depth and quality, image location, and special effects such as glows, sparkles, shimmers. Take each of these to its greatest intensity—for instance, the image could be increased to much greater than life-size. If this image were a god of that particular quality, how would these submodalities manifest? Just how big is a god/dess of *x*?

7. Begin to add in extra features and aspects from other humans, from animals, or from machines as appropriate to a god/dess of this quality. For instance, if cunning and strength are important to your highest aspirations, give it some qualities of a tiger or other animal that might represent those qualities (head, body, teeth, eyes, whatever). If enhanced intelligence or processing speed is important, then maybe a computer chip or having a computer as an accessory might work. Take as much time as is necessary to test out some of these qualities. Notice which ones feel the best and keep them. Have fun with this and make your image fantastic.

8. Adjust physiology to account for the additions. If you added a computer chip to the brain, how would that be reflected in facial expression, breathing, posture, etc.?

9. Contemplate the image for at least thirty seconds.

10. Take a deep breath and, as you exhale, send the god-image into the chalice of bhang. Say out loud, "I consecrate the contents of this chalice to [name of deity]."

11. Cover the chalice, wrap it in a piece of clean cloth (hemp if available), and place it in a special place until it is time to use it in ritual (soon, of course, while the milk is still good). The contents of the chalice are now considered soma.

GROUP CONSECRATION TO A META-DEITY

1. Have a bowl or chalice that is used only for consecrating or holding consecrated cannabis. Prepare a fresh batch of bhang to be consecrated and put it in the special chalice.

2. Participants sit in a circle and a banishing is performed to clear the space. This can be as simple as each participant practicing expansion/contraction breathing, filling and clearing the work area.

3. The group selects an objective or quality for which they would like to create a group-mind deity.

4. The elements of that objective or quality are identified. In a small group, each participant can suggest one element. In a larger group a fixed number can be agreed upon and suggestions can be ratified by consensus, vote, or decision-maker.

5. Each participant imagines a humanoid figure in the center of the circle and makes appropriate adjustments to the figure as the ritual proceeds.

6. Each participant, in turn, makes a suggestion concerning the physical attributes of the entity. These may concern the sex of the entity; its size, color, shape, posture, gestures, and facial features; number of limbs; special effects and features; and so on. Almost anything is fair game as long as it represents, in the mind of the suggesting participant, that objective, overall quality, or any of the elements. For instance, in seminars we have developed godforms with six arms, green skin, gills, sharp teeth, feline bodies, etc.

7. Participants simultaneously develop state entities for each of the chosen elements and place these into the group entity. For instance, if the

elements are speed, intelligence, and patience, then all participants will develop their own "speed" state entity and place it into the godform, then all will develop their own for intelligence and add them to the mix, then all will develop state entities for patience and place them into the godform.

8. Participants breathe into the godform and continue to offer the godform breath and attention through the remainder of the ritual.

   Each participant, in their own mind, asks the godform for one syllable of the god's name. When each has added their syllable, the sounds are combined to create the full name of the god/dess.

9. Everyone takes a deep breath and, as they exhale, sends the god-image into the chalice of bhang. Say together, out loud, "I consecrate the contents of this chalice to [name of deity]."

10. Cover the chalice, wrap it in a piece of clean cloth (hemp if available), and place it in a special place until it is time to use it in ritual (soon, of course, while the milk is still good). The contents of the chalice are now considered soma.

SACRIFICES AND OFFERINGS

Academics and magicians often debate the difference between sacrifice and offering. To simplify a bit, we'll use the following definitions here: Sacrifice is the act of giving something negative away. Something that impedes your progress, distracts from your practice, makes you a worse human being, or runs contrary to your higher aspirations is embodied and cast away. An offering, as we'll use the term here, is a positive act, something that is given to an entity, an ideal, or an aspiration that gives it energy, empowers it, feeds it, or makes it more possible. Think of these as similar to the ideas of yama and niyama in yoga, the "thou shalt nots" versus virtuous behavior.

Making a Sacrifice

1. Decide on what you can be rid of in order to come closer to your highest aspirations. For the most part, these are personal biases, habits, and

limiting beliefs. Sometimes the specifics may be obvious, other times you may need to be more general. For most of us, a bit of dishabituation is a good thing, so a general casting out of cultural conditioning might be the default position. If this is a group working, each individual can make their own sacrifice, or the group can decide on a quality/entity to sacrifice and everyone can do it together.

2. Embody the thing to be cast out. That is, give it at least temporary entityhood. For example, humorless prudery might be embodied by Grayface, whom we met earlier in the Discordian banishing. If it is easily done, give your sacrificial quality a shape, a face, and a name. If this is less obvious, you can use an "energy flow" process:

   a. Think about how your sacrificial quality feels to you or how you feel when you think about it.

   b. Notice what kind of feeling it is and where in your body you have the feeling.

   c. Assign a color or colors to the feeling; apply it everywhere in your body that you have the feeling.

   d. Take the colored shape out of your body and breathe into it.

   e. Use the colored shape/entity as your sacrifice.

3. Find a symbolic way to dispose of the sacrifice. Laugh at it until it disintegrates. Fire it on a rocket into the sun. Blow it up. Sink it in the deepest ocean. Tear it to shreds with your hands.

Making an Offering

1. Think about what factors you would like to call on to assist you in your highest aspirations. This can include ancestors, elemental spirits, opener entities (such as Legba or Atem), magical schools, traditions, egregores, deities you have worked with in the past, friends, forces of nature, familiars, and perhaps some of your own personality characteristics. Pick several of the most important ones and think of them as leaflets on a cannabis leaf.

2. Pour out a small amount of soma, onto the ground, into water, or into a symbolic vessel for each of these factors, naming each one as you do so and calling upon it to assist you. For instance, "I offer this to you, my ancestors, that you may assist me in my highest aspiration. Thank you for your assistance." (Use small, symbolic amounts of soma and make sure you save most of the soma for the main part of the ritual.)

BANISHING

As discussed elsewhere in this book, banishing in a high magick tradition is often more than just clearing out a space. Rituals such as the Lesser Banishing Ritual of the Pentagram or the Star Ruby are, in effect, miniature versions of a Holy Guardian Angel operation, a way to contact and identify with your "higher self" or true will. These rituals also provide a strong sense of orientation in space and time and, on the lattice of that orientation, a structure or shape for the submodalities of present consciousness.[143]

The banishing sets the stage for the invocation to come, so you want your rituals to match in some basics. It is helpful if the symbolism matches. If your invocation is based in qabala or astrology or alchemy, then choose a banishing that is compatible. If you work in a circle, then both rituals can be circular. And so on.

If you know a traditional or personal banishing ritual and feel comfortable working with that, this is the time to break it out. The traditional rituals often prove to be surprisingly elegant and packed with information and they are definitely worth the study. If you are not yet familiar with one of those, here's a simple leaf symbol banishing.

Lesser Banishing Ritual of the Leaf

1. Define the area in which you intend to work. Is it a circle? A room? An outdoor field?

2. Within that space, imagine a nine-pointed leaf. Stand at the place where the leaflets meet the stem.

---

143. Or, for the more mystically inclined, a shape for your aura.

3. For each of the leaf elements—soil, air, sun, roots, stalk, leaves, flowers, smoke, and seed—perform the following:

    a. At the tip of the leaflet, imagine a ball of energy that represents the element. Think about the general characteristics of the element—for instance, air might be cool, transparent, flowing, windy, etc.; sun can be hot, bright, radiating, etc.—and fill that ball of energy with the qualities.

    b. Imagine the energy of that element flowing out from the ball, sweeping through your area of working, filling it, and purifying it. Say the name of the element, loudly and clearly.

    c. Perform the same for the next leaflet and so on until all nine have been addressed.

4. Where you stand, imagine that you are getting larger. Imagine yourself as large as is practical in the space.

5. Imagine energy flowing into you from below, as if drawing it up from the earth via roots. Imagine energy flowing into you from above, as if absorbing energy from the sun. Imagine this energy feeding and empowering the energy centers of your body, your nervous system and chakras.

6. Walk to the edge of your working area and walk around the circumference, clockwise, three times, then return to your original position.

7. Shout, sing, bang a drum, or otherwise make some noise that fills up the working area, chasing out any contrary forces.

INVOCATION OF THE HIGHEST

Your own rituals and invocations will usually be the most effective at this point. If you have some idea of the nature of your highest aspiration, then speak to it, recite poetry, tell stories about it, display images that relate to it, play music, dance, drum, dream, smoke, or however else you would like to honor and make connection with your aspirations. The more exciting and compelling you make it, the better. At the climax of the invocation, all participants consume the soma.

If, however, you are still in the process of defining what that aspiration may be for you or are still getting comfortable with the idea of creating and practicing ritual, here is a basic invocation to start with.

Invocation

1. If available, place a live cannabis plant in the center of the working area. An imaginary plant will do if an actual one cannot be obtained. Take a moment and contemplate the plant. Understand the flow of life from seed and roots to flowers and the flowering of consciousness and civilization.

2. Imagine (or reinforce, if already used in the banishing) a nine-pointed leaf on the floor of your working area, filling the area.

3. At the tip of a leaflet, imagine that you see yourself standing, full of the properties of soil (or air, sun, roots, etc., in turn). Make the image of yourself at least life-size and eliminate any background from the image. Repeat for each leaflet and element. Remember that these are symbolic properties as well as literal ones:

    Soil—the basis, the raw materials, the ancestors

    Air—purification, catalysis, the elements that stoke the fire

    Sun—energy, will, fire, power to do things

    Roots—stability, transformation (of soil to nutrients), connections to others

    Stalk—strength, support, transport (of nutrients to cells)

    Leaves—interface with environment, transformation (of sun to growth)

    Flowers—culmination, harvest, thoughts, ideas, beauty, inspiration

    Smoke—physical transformation, death, aspiration, transience

    Seed—potential, start of a new cycle, thoughts of the future

4. Take a moment to look at the various versions of yourself at the tip of each leaflet. Notice how they differ. Notice how they stand, breathe, move, etc. Breathe into each one in turn and say its name (soil, air, etc.) loudly and clearly.

5. Imagine that the nine self-images walk toward you, converging into a single figure just in front of you. Notice how the images merge, notice what happens as they join with each other. Then have the figure turn around so that its back is toward you.

6. Step into the figure. Notice any feelings, thoughts, or ideas that come to you.

7. Drink the soma.

8. If possible, remain in the working area until the soma begins to have an effect. The time (which might be up to ninety minutes or more) can be spent continuing invocation, drumming, dancing, speaking out loud about highest aspirations, drawing images, recording your experiences, etc. If the time is not available, then continue on to the next ritual process.

TALISMANS AND ANCHORS

Once the deity or highest aspiration has been invoked, you can create talismans and anchors that you can use later to help recall the experience. If in the previous section you drew images or created artifacts of some kind, those can be used to create talismans. If you haven't, it's simple enough to create something at this point or to use an object that you consecrate to the purpose. The object chosen is best if it has some symbolic value relating to your aspiration. Crystals, amber, carvings, jewelry, images, coins, vessels, or almost anything else can be used as long as

a. the object has not been used for a similar purpose previously; and

b. from this point on, the object is only used for its talismanic quality and not for any mundane purpose.

Talisman Anchors

1. Notice how you feel following the invocation. Which feelings denote your highest aspiration?

2. Pay attention to those feelings. Note where in your body you feel them and what kind of feeling it might be (tingling, pressure, temperature, texture, or anything else).

3. Nurture those feelings and let them intensify and expand.

4. Give the feelings a color or colors.

5. Take a large toke from a joint or pipe and exhale the smoke along with the colors and the feelings toward the object you wish to work with. (If you don't want to smoke, you can take a small sip of soma and spit it at the object, though this is a messier process. An imaginary joint can also be employed.) Imagine the object absorbing the colors and feelings.

6. Wrap the object in a clean cloth (preferably hemp) and place it in a safe place until it is needed.

7. Later, to remind yourself of your highest aspiration or to enhance the power of that aspiration in yourself, you can hold the object, carry it in your pocket, or display it where it can be seen.

FUTURE PACING

The final part of almost any ritual is to look back at what was done in the ritual, to notice what has changed during the ritual, and to consider how it will affect your future. Reviewing and noticing changes is often best accomplished by journaling, making an entry in your magical record (if you keep one), or explaining out loud (and recording it, if possible). Remembering, even in the short term, can be thought of as "putting the pieces together," as the word suggests, in a way that builds a personal narrative. Contemplating the future is a function of imagination, though it is still about putting the pieces together and setting a basic form for narratives to come.

Remembering the Future

1. Take a few moments to recall this ritual, from the initial preparation through the creation of talismans. Remember what happened and how it felt, looked, sounded, tasted, and smelled.

2. Consider how it feels now, after drinking the soma and completing the ritual.

3. Think about some upcoming situations in your life. If these will benefit from the experience of your highest aspiration, so much the better.

4. Imagine how you will look, sound, and feel in those upcoming situations, with knowledge and experience of your highest aspiration. In these imaginings, think about how you will stand, sit, or lie, what your posture will be like, how you will breathe, what your facial expression will convey, and anything else that may express your aspirations. Consider, in your imagination, how other people will respond to you when you are in this state and any other kinds of benefits you think you may experience.

CLOSING THE RITUAL

This can be simple. If there are any imagined things still external to you, reabsorb them back into you. Take a walk around your working area, three times clockwise. Then declare the ritual ended, put away your tools, cover any remaining soma, and put it away (or drink it or pour it out).

SOME GENERAL TIPS

Think of these instructions as a general structure rather than a script. Create your own specifics, use your own art, music, and movement—or favorite and inspiring works by others. Make it flow, make it compelling, and make it memorable.

There is a tendency to make important rituals serious and boring. There may be times when the ritual is used for a solemn purpose and solemnity may be appropriate, but for the most part, this ritual works better as a celebration. Have fun. Keep your sense of humor. Use laughter when appropriate. Be serious about your outcomes and humorous in your methods.

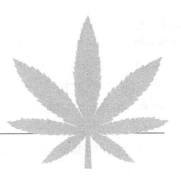

CHAPTER TWENTY-SEVEN

EVOLUTION

It is easy to track how humans have influenced the evolution and spread of the cannabis plant. Every strain that we know about is most likely a cultivar, something grown and bred by humans. As early humans discovered the healing, magical, and industrial qualities of the plant, we picked out the best examples and selectively bred for the traits that we found valuable.

It is more difficult to track the influence that the plant had on humans, but that influence is significant. Let's start with a little bit of speculation. Terence McKenna proposed his "stoned ape" theory in 1992, suggesting that entheogens including cannabis (and McKenna's favorite, psilocybin mushrooms) were a major influence in humanity's "great leap forward," the Paleolithic emergence of language, art, and culture. Mark Merlin and Robert C. Clarke in their massive textbook *Cannabis: Ethnobotany and Evolution* suggest that a random mutation in the CB1 receptor may have accelerated the evolution of human cognitive abilities. They theorize that early humans who sought food and fiber from cannabis came into contact with the psychoactive parts of the plant. Contact with the plant represented an evolutionary selective force favoring those with more cannabinoid receptors. For instance, cannabis was one of the very first plants woven into fabric (if not actually the first) and Merlin and Clarke propose that not only was the plant a source of fiber but also supported the intelligence and creativity necessary to conceive of crafts such as weaving.[144]

Weaving is only one of many survival-oriented skills associated with this plant of many uses. Those who improved their existence by eating nutritious seeds, using rope, or treating their illnesses with medicine would thrive and pass along their cannabis traditions to future generations. The more relaxed, nurturing, and less-aggressive mental states associated with cannabis may also be a survival trait as population increases and we have to live closer to and cooperate more with our neighbors.[145] As we've discussed, these choices and preferences may be passed down epigenetically—and genetically as well.

A 2007 study[146] gave intriguing evidence that the presence of cannabinoids speeds the evolution of the human nervous system. Studying the receptors and rates of gene mutation in both rats and humans, the researchers found that the CB1 receptors are evolving much more quickly in humans, with the suggestion that contact with plant cannabinoids may be driving rapid evolution of the human nervous system.

A physician who has worked extensively with medical marijuana patients, Dr. Robert Melamede, has another way of understanding the evolutionary properties of the endocannabinoid system. The CB1 receptors in the brain regulate energy metabolism and help to protect the brain from, in effect, burning out. The increased complexity of the human brain, relative to other vertebrates, requires more cannabinoid receptors, which suggests that people with more brain-power will be well-endowed with more cannabinoid receptors. Dr. Melamede sorts the human race into two broad categories: those with less or deficient receptor sites in the brain, whom he dubs "Backward Looking People" (BLP), and those with more receptor sites and more complex ways of thinking, whom he calls "Forward Looking People" (FLP). The BLPs tend to have simpler, linear, rigid thought patterns, while the FLPs tend to have looser, more open, and more imaginative thoughts. As the cannabis plant continues to

---

144. Clarke and Merlin, 2013.

145. Ibid.

146. McPartland et al. "Coevolution between Cannabinoid Receptors and Endocannabinoid Ligands." *Gene* 397, 2007.

spread and gain in acceptance worldwide, exposure to plant cannabinoids may help the FLPs increase in numbers and acceptance.[147]

In the famous nineteenth-century occult society the Golden Dawn, the goal of practicing high magick was to become "more than human." The suggestion was that magick and meditation could offer powers and abilities beyond the ordinary. While some of the touted skills may have been more wishful thinking than actuality—for instance, invisibility or levitation—modern science has corroborated the cognitive advantages and benefits of both ritual and meditation.

If Leary and Wilson were correct about their eight-circuit model of consciousness, then we are now observing, in some individuals, the emergence of new evolutionary functions of the human nervous system. Cannabis has certainly been a part of the emergence of the neurosomatic circuit, if only by making such experiences possible and giving humans a sample of what to strive for.

There's no question that worldwide use of the cannabis plant, as ancient and widespread as it may already be, continues to grow and become commonplace. This is an evolutionary success story for the plant and definitely an influence on the evolution of humans. As we face a future that includes the challenges of climate change, increased population, pollution, war, and everything else that humans struggle with, it will take imagination, creativity, compassion, and open minds for our species to thrive. Fortunately, we Forward Looking People know of a plant that might help.

147. Melamede, Robert. "BLPs and FLPs and Evolution." June 20, 2015. https://www.youtube.com/watch?v=HgzNptlY5zo.

MYTHBUSTING

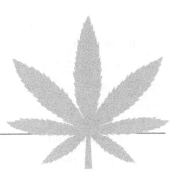

In our lifetime cannabis has been mostly illegal throughout the world. With only a few exceptions, the Netherlands being one of the most notable, nations have sought to appease or emulate the US, which enforces antidrug policies in all corners of the planet. How cannabis prohibition began is a bit hazy, but we know that several corporate and government entities supported the ban, including the US Department of the Treasury, the DuPont Corporation, Hearst newspapers, and others. Prohibition remains a boon for competing industries of synthetic textiles, wood-pulp paper, pharmaceuticals, alcohol, and tobacco, as well as a major source of funding for law enforcement and prisons.[148]

Not consulted on the move to ban cannabis in 1937—in fact, deliberately deceived about it—were the doctors. Doctors commonly prescribed cannabis tincture, but they had no clue what this evil drug "marijuana" might be and were surprised to find their cannabis removed from the shelves after the ban. A protest by the American Medical Association was ignored and the plant was demonized in every way possible.

Early attempts at anticannabis propaganda now seem corny and ridiculous. The hype was aimed at white racists who were led to believe that marijuana would tempt their daughters to attend wild parties where they would have sex

---

148. Gardner, Fred. "Who Orchestrated the Prohibition of Marijuana?" *Alternet*, July 25, 2013; Herer, Jack. *The Emperor Wears No Clothes: Hemp and the Marijuana Conspiracy*. AH HA Publishing, 2010.

with blacks and Mexicans. That kind of bullshit is now quite easy to spot; however, it has been largely replaced with a more subtle brand of bovine waste. You've read this far, so I'll assume you hold a more favorable opinion about weed, but even you—yes, even you—may still believe some of the silliness. So I often find that I must address a few common misconceptions.

Cannabis is physically bad for you (causes cancer, kills brain cells, warps your brain, makes men grow breasts, makes you fat, etc.). The theory that smoking weed would cause cancer was based on the presence of tars and combustion products in cannabis smoke similar to those found in carcinogenic tobacco smoke. However, long-term studies of cannabis smokers—even heavy smokers—have repeatedly found that they have less cancer than the general population and also less respiratory problems in general.[149] Not only does cannabis not kill brain cells, it appears to protect them from injury and even to stimulate the growth of new brain cells.[150] Studies examining long-term heavy cannabis users found that their brain structure was exactly the same as that of nonusers.[151] Yes, cannabis can make you feel hungry and frequent users will consume, on average, six hundred calories per day more than nonusers—but we still stay leaner, have better glucose metabolism, and less diabetes.[152] And no, it doesn't make men grow breasts.

Cannabis makes you lazy. Propagandists like to use the big term "amotivational syndrome" to make this sound more authoritative, but it's just not true. This was first debunked in the 1970s in a long-term study of cannabis-using Jamaican farm workers—who produced more than their nonusing peers.[153] A somewhat sadistic Canadian study, also in the '70s, locked a group of

---

149. Tashkin, Ribeiro L. "Marijuana and the lung: hysteria or cause for concern?" *Breathe,* 2018, 196–205.

150. Jiang et al. "Cannabinoids promote embryonic and adult hippocampus neurogenesis and produce anxiolytic-and antidepressant-like effects." *The Journal of Clinical Investigation.* 2005.

151. Martin-Santos et al. "Neuroimaging in cannabis use: a systematic review of the literature," *Psychological Medicine,* Volume 40, Issue 3, March 2010.

152. Penner et al. "The Impact of Marijuana Use on Glucose, Insulin, and Insulin Resistance among US Adults." *The American Journal of Medicine.* Volume 126, Issue 7, 2013.

153. Rubin, Vera, and Lambros Comitas. *Ganja in Jamaica: A Medical Anthropological Study of Chronic Marihuana Use.* Mouton De Gruyter, 1975.

women in a laboratory and made them smoke increasingly stronger doses of cannabis every day while producing handmade crafts for pay on commission. While many of the women dropped out because of the sheer lunacy of the experiment, the conclusion, long suppressed by the Canadian government, was that cannabis use had no effect on productivity. A 2016 study of residents in California and Colorado, where cannabis is legal, showed that, across the board, cannabis users had higher-paying jobs, more employment in general, a higher level of education, a tendency to volunteer more, more sex, and rated their lives as being more satisfying.[154] And, in general, cannabis use crosses through broad cultural lines, with highly successful businessmen, Olympic athletes, presidents of the US, famous scientists, and plenty of other highly motivated and high-profile people all as likely to puff up as anyone else.[155]

Cannabis makes you crazy. Ha ha! Maybe it does, but only if we go by a very narrow definition of sanity. In recent years, government-sponsored agencies have churned out a variety of poorly conceived studies showing a correlation between cannabis use and psychosis. All of those studies, or at least the headlines derived from them, ignore the statistical axiom that "correlation does not equal causality," and at least one of the studies also demonstrated that psychosis was a predicting factor for later cannabis use. Seems simple to me; people who feel bad find an effective way to self-medicate. To say that cannabis causes psychosis is much like claiming that because millions of headache sufferers take aspirin, aspirin must cause headaches! Indeed, there is a similar correlation between schizophrenia and cigarette use (nicotine also seems to temporarily alleviate some symptoms), but I haven't yet heard the claim that tobacco causes schizophrenia. Studies in which cannabis was given to schizophrenic patients demonstrated that it helped improve their

154. Brown, Doug. "Cannabis Consumers are Happy Campers," *BDS Analytics*. June 6, 2016. http://bdsanalytics.com/cannabis-consumers-happy-campers/.

155. Komp, Ellen. "Very Important Potheads: Changing the Face of Cannabis," 2001–2019. http://www.veryimportantpotheads.com/; Bob, "The 10 Smartest Pot Smokers on the Planet Cool Enough to Admit it," *COED*, November, 2016. http://coed.com/2011/02/02/the-10-smartest-pot-smokers-on-the-planet-cool-enough-to-admit-it/.

cognitive abilities and function in general.[156] A Harvard University study adds support to the role of genetic factors in schizophrenia and states that marijuana use alone does not increase the risk of developing the disorder. The latest findings provide enough evidence for Dr. DeLisi and her team to conclude that "Cannabis is unlikely to be the cause of this illness."[157] The use of cannabinoids to treat psychosis has aroused the interest of the pharmaceutical industry, and at least one company is now developing a cannabinoid antipsychotic medication.[158]

Cannabis has no medical use. This is what government agencies in several countries maintain, even while licensing cannabis drugs from pharmaceutical companies and ignoring clinical trials and research originating from more enlightened nations. Clinical evidence mounts for the effective use of cannabis in multiple sclerosis, Crohn's disease, neuropathy, muscle spasticity, and treatment of cancer. In the U.S.A., where some states allow medical cannabis, there is an idea that only the most seriously sick should have access to it. I'm not sure why that is—cannabis has a better safety profile than most over-the-counter medications, including aspirin. People die from taking aspirin, sometimes, but no one ever dies as a direct result of taking cannabis. And it is very good for common aches, pains, headaches, migraines, insomnia, even hemorrhoids.

Today's pot is stronger than the old stuff. No. Wrong again. Please don't misunderstand me; there is some killer bud to be had today and the excellent stuff is certainly easier to get. But there was great weed years ago, too. And I'm not just talking about a few decades; I'm talking about history, about thousands of years of kick-ass cannabis. The historic strains of weed are still around, grown by hobbyists and horticulturists. That includes the ones from decades ago, things like Thai Stick, Santa Marta Gold, Acapulco Gold, Pan-

---

156. Armentano, Paul. "Debunking the Myth of a Link Between Marijuana and Mental Illness." *Alternet*, July 25, 2011. https://www.alternet.org/story/151776/debunking_the_myth_of_a_link_between_marijuana_and_mental_illness.

157. Proal et al. "A controlled family study of cannabis users with and without psychosis." *Schizophrenia Research*, Volume 152, Issue 1, July 2014.

158. McGuire et al. "Cannabidiol (CBD) as an Adjunctive Therapy in Schizophrenia: A Multicenter Randomized Controlled Trial." *American Journal of Psychiatry*, March 2018.

ama Red, Durban Poison, and so forth. And modern farmers have tested the cannabinoids in these strains and they are just as potent as good dispensary weed. In fact, much of today's ganja, "skunk" for instance, was bred from those famous golds and reds. And the strains from the dawn of cannabis history—some of those are still around, too. There are Nepali strains that may be the mothers of all sativa plants, cultivated for thousands of years on the slopes of the Himalayas. That stuff is over 15 percent THC, which is pretty kick-ass, as good as most of the ganja for sale in the US. Malawi cannabis that has been grown for hundreds of years, at least, by the same farmers on the same land in Africa tests at around 18 percent THC. That's strong weed! Some Central Asian varieties, in the mountains where cannabis is thought to have originated, top 20 percent THC, which is at the very high end for any kind of ganja. By comparison, the average potency for black market weed in the US is around 9 percent, and good dispensary bud is more often in the 12 to 20 percent range. It's true that back in the day there was a lot of awful stuff for sale to an ignorant market. Schwag. Bunkweed. Dirtweed. Some of it was rope hemp from abandoned farms, but most of it probably began life as good bud and then, through time and poor treatment, got moldy, lost potency, began to compost, and generally turned to shit. But anyone with a good connection and a nose for quality could get the good stuff, too, and it didn't cost much more, back then. Now it costs a whole lot more. The whole concept of out-of-control potency is designed to make us think that somehow the weed gets more dangerous as it gets more potent. It does not. Actually, I wish cannabis today were more potent. More potent is good! It allows you to titrate your dose and smoke less.[159]

Cannabis is addictive. People use that word, "addictive," but I do not think they know what it means. There's a neuropharmacological experience of addiction that has to do with the release of dopamine in the brain. There are a lot of drugs that cause that, from coffee to heroin. But cannabis isn't on that list. In fact, recent studies demonstrate that it tends to lower dopamine levels a little bit. Of course, some people misuse it and develop compulsions

---

159. Holland, 2010.

or habits concerning cannabis. These are the same kinds of compulsions that we might develop for a favorite TV show, rock band, stamp collection, comic books, web surfing, video games, or whatever it is that fascinates us. When these compulsions get in the way of work, relationships, and so on (as all the above examples have the potential to do), then that is a problem. But it's not the same thing as a physiological addiction and requires a different kind of treatment. Some of these compulsive people claim withdrawal symptoms when they stop using cannabis, usually irritability or sleep problems. As withdrawal symptoms go, these are incredibly mild, and I don't really believe they are actual withdrawal symptoms. More likely they are preexisting problems that were being treated by the cannabis! In my case, I am a teacher of cannabis magick! I smoke every day, when I'm working. But sometimes I have to travel or otherwise be in situations where I cannot have any ganja for days or even weeks at a time. I have never, ever noticed anything like withdrawal symptoms. There are statistics out there showing how many people go to rehab for "cannabis addiction," and it's an impressive number—however, most of those who go to rehab for cannabis do it because they are ordered to by a court, not because they believe they have an addiction.[160]

Remember! This historical period of anticannabis hype is a blip (and the product of BLPs), an aberration in human history. For ten thousand years, cannabis was not only accepted in most parts of the world but revered as well. Less than a hundred years of prohibition is nothing to this plant. Cannabis will adapt and endure and humans will once again learn of the symbiosis their ancestors enjoyed with this useful plant.

---

160. Ibid.

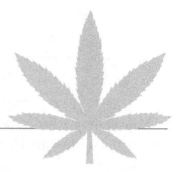

DANGERS

OVERDOSE, PARANOIA, PANIC

Let me begin by reminding you that cannabis is, indeed, one of the safest substances known to man. The lethal dose of it is so very high (ha ha!) that it would be improbable that anyone could actually ingest that much. There are no known deaths caused directly by smoking or eating cannabis. Some unpleasant situations, yes, but no one dies, and everyone feels better in the morning.

If we define an overdose as "more than I wanted to take," then, sure, it's possible to overdose and have a bad time. This is more common, as I mentioned earlier, when eating cannabis, which makes titration difficult. Eating or smoking too much can, in rare cases, prompt a freakout, but mostly it means a good long sleep followed by a few hours of grogginess.

But, yes, freakouts do happen and not always because someone takes too much. See the discussion on "set and setting" for more specifics, but in general, figure there are times and places when it's just not comfortable or sane to get high. In places where it is still illegal, for instance, paranoia can become a big issue. THC causes arousal in the brain and heightened perception, and if you are worried about getting busted, those are the thoughts that will be heightened and every little sound or movement will seem like a narcotics officer lurking outside the window.

Sometimes, very strong ganja from high THC strains will cause tachycardia. That means that your heart will race and pound for a minute or two. While this is generally harmless (if you have a heart condition and worry about such things, then your worry is probably enough reason to avoid the experience), for some people it is physiologically similar to the onset of a panic attack. If it is similar enough, then it can, potentially, trigger an attack. If this happens to you or to a friend, be reassured that it is simply a minor physiological effect of something you ingested; breathe deeply (and sit with your back straight!) a few times and it will pass quickly. Certain aromas can also interact with cannabis in ways that help to induce calm, most notably black pepper, lemons, or oranges. And get your panic attacks checked out by a doctor, too!

If paranoia and panic are persistent, you might explore changing to a different strain of ganja with a higher CBD content or more relaxing range of terpenes, combining your smoking sessions with yogic breathing exercises, or simply avoiding cannabis until you have resolved these issues in your life. Come back to it another time, when you will enjoy it and profit from it more.

Similarly, some people have different body chemistry or neurological predispositions and simply do not enjoy cannabis. If they try it and are particularly uncomfortable, the same advice applies: remind them that it is something that they consumed, it is harmless and it will pass soon enough. They might, at another time, try a different kind of cannabis, or simply abstain. While most people can find benefit from cannabis, it's not for everyone.

TOO MUCH

As I mentioned before, there are some people who become compulsive and do too much. Don't get me wrong, in general I have no qualms about daily use or even constant use, in the right setting, for the right people. However, there are an inevitable few in any activity who get obsessed or take it too far. When ganja use (or TV, net porn, video games, occult books, etc.) interferes with basic survival, it's a problem. If you spend the rent money on ganja and then get evicted, you're not managing your life properly. If you get fired from your job for smoking or showing up too stoned, you are probably doing too much. If you cease to work for the goals and dreams of your life, you need to reexamine everything you do, cannabis use included. If you are obsessed with getting high to the point where you do not bathe or clean up after yourself and you get sick as a result, that's a problem and you need help managing your life, time, and personal hygiene. In general, we must remember that our intent in smoking is more important than the smoke itself. Do we do it to make sex better, give devotion to our god, create art, heal ourselves, enhance perception, or wax philosophic? Or do we do it as an end in itself that is more important than the direction and purpose of our lives? Just remember that ganja is, among other things, a tool. What we do with a tool is usually more important than the tool itself.

If, however, frequent use honestly benefits what you do in your life, and promotes health, reason, and spirituality, then I will say, "More power to you!"

CRAPPY WEED

Yes, crappy weed is a danger, perhaps the biggest danger to the casual, medical, or ritual smoker. Because cannabis is often available only through an unregulated black market, some dealers are pretty shady. Do you think a cartel gangster in another country has your health and well-being in mind? Poorly treated cannabis can be as dangerous as poorly treated food. Really, you don't want to ingest mold, bacteria, pesticides, and chemical contaminants in your weed any more than you do in your dinner. Mold and bacteria in smoked cannabis can cause bronchitis and other chronic conditions, as well as acute allergic reactions. A precaution that you can take is to heat your cannabis at 150 degrees Fahrenheit for five minutes to help kill contaminants. However, if you see that there is obvious mold or mildew on your buds, or if they smell musty, then throw the shit out and do not, in any way, ingest it, no matter how much you paid for it or how much effort you expended growing it. Mold can cause serious lung conditions and worse.

Some growers are less scrupulous than others and will pump chemical fertilizers into their plants without flushing them out thoroughly prior to harvest. Properly grown cannabis will burn to a mostly pure white or very light gray ash. Cannabis with fertilizer residue will leave black bits or the ash will be mostly black, no matter how much you torch it. Think twice about smoking unflushed weed.

Even worse, some larger and, again, unscrupulous growers will use pesticides on the buds. It's hard to tell if they have, so the solution here is to only purchase your ganja from known and trusted sources, from dispensaries and shops that test weed for purity, or to grow it yourself.

Less common, but it still occasionally happens: someone will adulterate herbal cannabis with psychoactive chemicals of various sorts. Back a few decades ago, it was often PCP, known as angel dust, though I have also seen cannabis adulterated with heroin and other opiates, synthetic cannabinoids, *salvia divinorum*, and various other psychoactive chemicals and herbs. The unscrupulous part of this comes with lack of disclosure. If you know there's something in your bag of weed and choose to do it in an informed way, I can't argue with you. But getting a chemical surprise when you expect a nice cannabis experience is annoying and, indeed, possibly very dangerous.

As with any other ritual tool, you want to make sure your cannabis represents the integrity and quality with which you perform your magick.

SIDE EFFECTS AND DRUG INTERACTIONS

Yes, there are a few side effects to ganja. The most dangerous of them is orthostatic hypotension. That's a fancy term for the head rush you get when you stand up too fast, which can be greatly magnified by certain kinds of cannabis. If you think you've got that kind of buzz going, stand up slowly. Sit back down if it gets too much. Breathe. It will pass and apart from the possibility of falling over, it is harmless.

Other side effects include dry mouth, red eyes, and hunger. None of these are dangerous in any way. Drink plenty of fluids and have healthy snacks on hand.

Cannabis may interact with other herbs and drugs. Smoked with tobacco, as it often is in Europe, cannabis can exacerbate respiratory damage and may lead to nicotine addiction. Combined with alcohol, coordination may be considerably more impaired than with alcohol alone. On the other hand, cannabis seems to provide some protection against the neurological damage caused by alcohol.[161] Let's just say you'll be a little more wasted but perhaps healthier in the morning.

Do you take any medications that have a "grapefruit warning" on them? It is well-known that grapefruit affects the metabolism of some drugs, either increasing their effects or inhibiting them, depending on the substance. Cannabis that is high in CBD may have a similar effect as grapefruit. So, if (a) your medication has a grapefruit warning, and (b) you have cannabis that is high in CBD, combine carefully and in very small quantities, if at all, until you know what kind of interaction there might be. Even better, ask your doctor about it.

Cannabis seems to have some synergy with opiates, as well, which is a boon for chronic pain patients who may choose to take less narcotics, but, again, impairment of coordination may be greater than anticipated. Cannabis may also intensify the befuddling and sedative effects of other central nervous system depressants, and some antihistamines. Combine carefully and you know how it goes: do not drive or operate heavy machinery until you know how the drugs affect you.

A few common pharmaceuticals and nutrients may reduce or inhibit aspects of the cannabis high. Ibuprofen may reduce the amount of short-term memory disruption produced by cannabis.[162] This is useful if you are very high and suddenly find yourself in a situation where greater continuous focus is required, though in general, the short-term memory effects of cannabis are half the fun. The prohormone pregnenolone, often available from vitamin and food supplement vendors, may diminish the high as well.[163]

Terpene-rich herbs and fruit may increase or decrease some of the effects of cannabis. Most well-known in this regard is the ability of mangoes to intensify or prolong a cannabis experience. Yes, it's true; if you eat a mango about one hour before getting high, you'll find that you can get a little higher for an

161. Liput et al. "Transdermal delivery of cannabidiol attenuates binge alcohol-induced neurodegeneration in a rodent model of an alcohol use disorder." *Pharmacology Biochemistry and Behavior*, Volume 111, October 2013.

162. Chen et al. "Δ⁹-THC-Caused Synaptic and Memory Impairments Are Mediated through COX-2 Signaling." *Cell*, Volume 155, Issue 5, November 2013.

163. Busquets-Garcia et al. "Pregnenolone blocks cannabinoid-induced acute psychotic-like states in mice." *Molecular Psychiatry*, February 2017.

hour or so longer than you usually would. Herbs such as wild thyme, lavender, and lemongrass also contain aromatic terpene chemicals that can potentially pump up the potency of your pot. Citrus oils, on the other hand, seem to reduce the intensity of the cannabis high and a big glass of lemonade or orange juice is a recommended antidote for an unpleasant cannabis experience.

For the most part, humans and cannabis have evolved together over the history of both our species. Millennia of cannabis use have proven our mutual adaptation and the safe use of the plant. We've selectively bred ganja that is not only safe but often beneficial, and cannabis has helped the human race survive, grow, and transform in numerous ways.

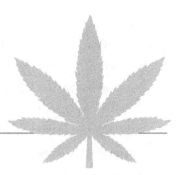

A FEW WORDS
ABOUT WORDS

C annabis has so many monikers that it is difficult to address them all. In the US, the most familiar name is marijuana, a Mexican term that was used by prohibitionists to rally racists against the herb. However, that word itself may have roots that are more interesting.

The most often cited origin for the term is "mariguan," first described by John G. Bourke in 1894, which referred to an herb used by women along the Rio Grande river for casting revenge spells and for receiving prophetic visions. As the revenge spells were likely not really spells but surreptitious poisoning, it may be more likely that this plant was not cannabis but *datura*, a poisonous deliriant also used, in much smaller doses, to induce visions.[164]

A somewhat better theory, in my opinion, is based on the presence of Chinese laborers in western Mexico. The Chinese word for hemp is *Ma* and various modifying syllables specify the different uses and parts of the plant. *Ma hua* refers to cannabis flowers. *Ma ren* means cannabis seed. And *Ma ren hua* would mean seeded flowers, the form of cannabis most common in Mexico up until recent times. An adaptation of that into Spanish could easily become marijuana, which means "Mary Jane." A slang term for cannabis that persisted

---

164. Piper, Alan. "'The Mysterious Origins of the Word 'Marijuana.'" *Sino-Platonic Papers*, Number 153, July 2005.

in Mexico over many years was Oregano Chino, or Chinese Oregano, perhaps attesting to the Chinese connection.[165]

It is likely that the Chinese root word Ma was the origin of many of the other historic terms we find for cannabis, including haoma (a reversal, perhaps, of the syllables *ma hua*), and soma (*sau ma* translates as "good hemp").[166]

It's tough to say who had the word *cannabis* first. The Assyrians called their herb *qunnabu*; in Persian it is *kenab*; *kannab* in Arabic; *kanbun* in Chaldean; *kaneh bosm* in ancient Hebrew; and *canna* in Sanskrit.[167] Certainly, the Scythians were the ones who spread their word *Kannabis* throughout Asia and Europe. Following the Scythians, it evolved into the Polish *konop*, Dutch *canvas*, Russian *konoplya*, Lithuanian *canapés*, Irish *canaib*, and so forth. In early European history, the "k" sound shifted to an "h" in many languages, yielding the Middle Low German *hennep*, modern German *hanf*, Swedish *hampa*, Anglo-Saxon *henep*, and the English *hemp*.[168]

The word hashish, commonly used to describe preparations of cannabis resin, is an Arabic term that simply means "grass."[169]

"Pot" most likely comes from the Spanish *potaguaya,* which is from the same root as our word *potion*.[170]

"Ganja" is a Sanskrit word for cannabis, carried all over the planet by sadhus and Rastas. The origin of the word is lost in antiquity but may have a connection to the river Ganges, where wild cannabis still grows today. Incredible healing properties are attributed to the waters of the river, a reputation earned, perhaps, in the distant past from the healing herb found there. The river, in turn, is personified by the goddess Ganga, who represents the flow of water and healing energy.

We typically use the words "high" and "stoned" to denote the cannabis experience. Some users will use "high" to refer to the headier kinds of high-THC

165. Ibid.

166. Bennett, 2010.

167. Benet, 1975.

168. Bennett, 2010.

169. Ibid.

170. "Is Marijuana Pot?" *GreenCulturED*. https://www.greencultured.co/is-marijuana-pot/.

herb and "stoned" to refer to the more narcotic varieties. "Stoned" comes from alcohol terminology, beginning as "stone drunk." For instance, the well-known Ray Charles song "Let's Get Stoned" is about drinking, not herb. Mostly, though, no one applies it to alcohol anymore. "High" is slightly more interesting, and while I can find no information on who first used the term, we can speculate. Many strains of cannabis produce a floating feeling that might be "high." We also use the term to describe a variety of spiritual and religious phenomena. God is the Most High. New agers seek their higher selves. Being ethical is described as taking the high road or the higher ground.

We can also think of "high" as a submodality term, a way that we describe the positioning of our internal representations that lets us know they are spiritual, better, more ethical, etc.

Some people consider both "high" and "stoned" to have too much connotation of "recreational" use or parallel to alcohol mentality. There aren't many alternative terms, so I've mostly used "high" in this volume. However, when I asked friends about terms that might be used to describe the more spiritual or meditative effects of cannabis, the brilliant DJ Reese suggested "sanctified." Get sanctified!

MAY YOUR SANCTIFICATION BRING HAPPINESS, HEALTH, AND ENLIGHTENMENT!

GLOSSARY

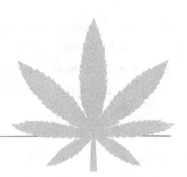

Anchor: The sensory stimuli that prompts the recall of a memory, behavior, or experience.

Avesta: The sacred texts of the Zoroastrian religion. Sometimes called the *Zend-Avesta*.

Banishing: A ritual act intended to prepare a space—and the magician—for further ritual.

Cannabinoids: The chemicals found in cannabis and the human body, including THC, CBD, and Anandamide, that bind to cannabinoid receptors. Phytocannabinoids are the ones found in the cannabis plant; endocannabinoids are found in the human body.

Chillum: A traditional straight smoking pipe used by sadhus and Rastas, among others.

Default Network: A network of brain systems that link up and process memories when conscious attention is not otherwise directed. The default network is responsible for daydreaming, spacing out, and transderivational search, among much else.

Endocannabinoid System (ECS): The system of receptor sites in the human body that acts as a master control, moderating homeostasis and many other physiological processes. The ECS maintains balance between the many systems in the body.

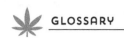

Evocation: The act of moving an idea, state, feeling, quality, or memory into a metaphoric position outside the body.

Executive Function: The opposite of the default network; the network of brain systems that allows for focused attention and problem solving in the moment.

Haoma: The ancient sacrament of the Avestan religions.

Holon: Anything that can symbolically represent a whole; a microcosm.

Indo-Europeans: An ancient people who spoke a common language and spread the soma sacrament throughout Asia and Europe.

Indra: A god who appears in Hinduism, Buddhism, and other religions. Indra is king of heaven and the heavenly deities. He was probably brought to India by the Indo-Europeans and his sacrament was the moon-plant used to make soma, probably cannabis.

Invocation: The act of drawing an idea, state, feeling, quality, or memory into a metaphoric position inside the body.

Khidr: A cannabis spirit revered by the Sufis, sometimes identified with the prophet Elijah.

Kundalini: The "Serpent Power" that lies coiled at the base of the spine, which can be aroused through meditation and yoga practices.

Magick: The art and science of causing change in conformity with Will.

Ma Gu: The Hemp Maiden, one of the Taoist immortals.

NLP: Neurolinguistic programming, the study of the structure of subjective experience.

Ritual Frame: Behaviors and symbols that mark out a period of time and everything within that time as being dedicated to a particular ritual goal.

Scythians: Nomadic horsemen who conquered a large part of Europe, Asia, and the Middle East from the ninth century BC to the fourth century AD.

Shiva: One of the principal deities of Hinduism, Lord of Yoga and Lord of Bhang.

Sigil: A pictorial symbol that represents the magician's intended outcome.

Soma: A sacrament used in the ancient world by Indo-Europeans, Scythians, Indians, and others. While different plants were used in various times and places, the original plant was probably cannabis.

Transderivational Search: The tendency of the mind to quickly sort a range of options when attempting to make sense of words and other sensory experiences. Transderivational search appears to be mediated by the brain's default network.

Terpene/Terpenoid: The aromatic chemicals that give cannabis and many other herbs their characteristic smells and flavors.

True Will: In Aleister Crowley's system of Thelema, true will is the term used to describe the unique purpose and direction of an individual.

Vedas: The sacred texts of Hinduism.

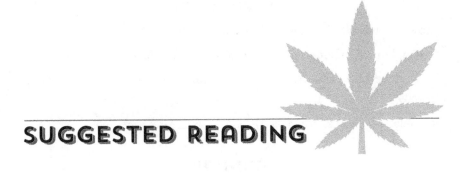

SUGGESTED READING

MAGICK

DuQuette, Lon Milo. *The Chicken Qabalah of Rabbi Lamed Ben Clifford.* Weiser Books, 2001.

DuQuette, Lon Milo. *The Magick of Aleister Crowley, a Handbook of the Rituals of Thelema.* Weiser Books, 2003.

Farber, Philip H. *Brain Magick: Exercises in Meta-Magick and Invocation.* Llewellyn, 2011.

Kraig, Donald M. *Modern Magick: Twelve Lessons in the High Magickal Arts.* Llewellyn, 2010.

HISTORY

Bennett, Chris. *Cannabis and the Soma Solution.* Trine Day, 2010.

Bennett, Chris. *Liber 420: Cannabis, Magical Herbs, and the Occult.* Trine Day, 2018.

Clarke, Robert, and Mark Merlin. *Cannabis: Evolution and Ethnobotany.* University of California Press, 2016.

Ratsch, Christian. *Marijuana Medicine: A World Tour of the Healing and Visionary Powers of Cannabis.* Healing Arts Press, 2001.

DIVINATION

Crowley, Aleister. *The Book of Thoth.* Samuel Weiser, 2011.

I-Ming, Lui, and Thomas Cleary. *The Taoist I Ching.* Shambhala, 2005.

Place, Robert M. *The Tarot: History, Symbolism, and Divination.* TarcherPerigee, 2005.

Randolph, P. B. *Seership and the Magic Mirror.* CreateSpace, 2008.

CANNABIS

Earleywine, Mitch. *Understanding Marijuana: A New Look at the Scientific Evidence.* Oxford University Press, 2002.

Gaskin, Stephen. *Cannabis Spirituality.* High Times, 1998.

Grinspoon, Lester, and James B. Bakalar. *Marihuana: The Forbidden Medicine.* Yale University Press, 1997.

Holland, Julie (ed.). *The Pot Book: A Complete Guide to Cannabis.* Park Street Press, 2010.

EIGHT-CIRCUIT MODEL OF CONSCIOUSNESS

Alli, Antero. *The Eight Circuit Brain: Navigational Strategies for the Energetic Body.* Original Falcon Press, 2017.

Wilson, Robert Anton. *Prometheus Rising.* Hilaritas Press, 2016.

ENTHEOGENS

Brown, David Jay. *The New Science of Psychedelics: At the Nexus of Culture, Consciousness, and Spirituality.* Park Street Press, 2013.

Hofmann, Albert, and Richard Evans Schultes. *Plants of the Gods: Their Sacred, Healing, and Hallucinogenic Powers.* Healing Arts Press, 2001.

Vayne, Julian. *Getting Higher: A Manual of Psychedelic Ceremony.* Psychedelic Press, 2017.

Weil, Andrew. *The Natural Mind: A Revolutionary Approach to the Drug Problem.* Mariner Books, 2004.

YOGA

Crowley, Aleister. *Eight Lectures on Yoga*. New Falcon, 1985.

Dussault, Dee. *Ganja Yoga: A Practical Guide to Conscious Relaxation, Soothing Pain Relief, and Enlightened Self-Discovery*. Hay House Publishing, 2017.

Iyengar, B.K.S. *Light on Pranayama: The Yogic Art of Breathing*. Crossroad Publishing, 1985.

Patanjali. *The Yoga Sutras of Patanjali*. Translated and with commentary by Swami Satchidananda. Integral Yoga Publications, 2012.

HYPNOSIS & NLP

Andreas, Steven, and Connirae Andreas. *Change Your Mind and Keep the Change: Advanced NLP Submodalities Interventions*. Real People Press, 1987.

Bandler, Richard. *Richard Bandler's Guide to TranceFormations: How to Harness the Power of Hypnosis to Ignite Effortless and Lasting Change*. HCI, 2008.

Bandler, Richard. *Using Your Brain for a Change: Neuro-linguistic Programming*. Real People Press, 1985.

LeCron, Leslie M. *Self Hypnotism: The Technique and Its Use in Daily Living*. Pearson, 1980.

LAUGHTER

Carlin, George. *Napalm and Silly Putty*. Hachette Books, 2002.

Farber, Philip H. *Legendary Blue Smoke*. Hoo-Ha Books, 2014.

Krassner, Paul. *Pot Stories for the Soul*. Soft Skull Press, 2012.

Malaclypse the Younger and Omar Khayyam Ravenhurst. *Principia Discordia*. CreateSpace, 2011.

Subgenius Foundation. *The Book of the SubGenius*. Touchstone, 1987.

INDEX

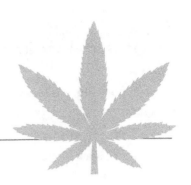

TO WRITE TO THE AUTHOR

If you wish to contact the author or would like more information about this book, please write to the author in care of Llewellyn Worldwide Ltd. and we will forward your request. Both the author and publisher appreciate hearing from you and learning of your enjoyment of this book and how it has helped you. Llewellyn Worldwide Ltd. cannot guarantee that every letter written to the author can be answered, but all will be forwarded. Please write to:

Philip H. Farber
℅ Llewellyn Worldwide
2143 Wooddale Drive
Woodbury, MN 55125-2989

Please enclose a self-addressed stamped envelope for reply,
or $1.00 to cover costs. If outside the U.S.A., enclose
an international postal reply coupon.

Many of Llewellyn's authors have websites with additional information and resources. For more information, please visit our website at http://www.llewellyn.com.